The WHEEL of
HEALING with
AYURVEDA

The WHEEL of HEALING with AYURVEDA

An Easy Guide to a Healthy Lifestyle

MICHELLE S. FONDIN

FOREWORD BY SUDHA BULUSU AND
DR. SHEKHAR ANNAMBHOTLA

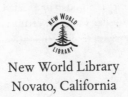

New World Library
Novato, California

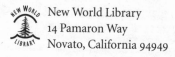

New World Library
14 Pamaron Way
Novato, California 94949

The material in this book is intended for education. It is not meant to take the place of diagnosis and treatment by a qualified medical practitioner or therapist. No expressed or implied guarantee of the effects of the use of the recommendations can be given nor liability taken.

Originally published in a different form as *The Wheel of Healing* in 2014.

Text design by Tona Pearce Myers

Library of Congress Cataloging-in-Publication Data
Fondin, Michelle S., date.
The wheel of healing with ayurveda : an easy guide to a healthy lifestyle / Michelle S. Fondin.
    pages   cm
Includes bibliographical references and index.
ISBN 978-1-60868-352-9 (paperback) — ISBN 978-1-60868-353-6 (ebook)
1. Medicine, Ayurvedic—Popular works. I. Title.
R605.F66 2015
615.5'38—dc23   2015001783

First printing, May 2015
ISBN 978-1-60868-352-9
Printed in Canada on 100% postconsumer-waste recycled paper

 New World Library is proud to be a Gold Certified Environmentally Responsible Publisher. Publisher certification awarded by Green Press Initiative. www.greenpressinitiative.org

10   9   8   7   6   5   4   3   2   1

Thirty spokes are joined together in a wheel,
but it is the center hole that allows the wheel to function.

— TAO TE CHING

CONTENTS

FOREWORD BY SUDHA BULUSU AND
    DR. SHEKHAR ANNAMBHOTLA   xi

ACKNOWLEDGMENTS   xv

PREFACE: My Story   xvii

INTRODUCTION: Reinventing the Wheel?   1

    Why the Wheel?   5
    Taking Back Your Health and Your Life   6
    Taking Responsibility for Your Health   8
    Exercise: Your Commitment to Yourself   9

CHAPTER 1. A Quick Immersion in Ayurveda   11

    What Is Ayurveda?   11
    Balance versus Imbalance   13
    The Ayurvedic Definition of Health   13
    The Mahabhutas: The Great Elements   14
    An Introduction to the Doshas   15
    The Ayurvedic Mind-Body Type Test   16
    Interpreting Your Mind-Body Type   25
    The Six Stages of Disease   27
    Creating a Symptom Plan   31
    Exercise: Identifying Your Typical Symptoms   32
    Checklist for Health: An Introduction to Ayurveda   32

CHAPTER 2. The Entire Wheel: Living Your Dharma,
    or Life's Purpose   33

    The Importance of Dharma   34
    Defining Dharma   35

Finding Your Dharma   39

Exercise: Discovering Dharma   40

Intention and Desire: Creating Your Life's Purpose   44

Exercise: List of Intentions and Desires   47

Checklist for Health: Dharma   48

CHAPTER 3. Physical Health   49

Food as Medicine   49

An Ayurvedic Plan for Optimal Nutrition   57

The Twelve Guidelines for an Ayurvedic Lifestyle Eating Plan   58

Guidelines for Re-creating the Mind-Body Connection with Food   70

Ten Guidelines for Eating Awareness   71

Eating for Your Mind-Body Type   74

Exercise: Your Dosha-Specific Eating Plan   78

Daily Routine and Seasonal Routine: Respecting Nature's Waves   80

Moving Your Body   86

Exercise: Creating Your Physical Movement Plan   90

Checklist for Health: Physical Healing   91

CHAPTER 4. Spiritual Health   93

What Defines Spiritual?   93

Embracing Your Spiritual Self   95

Going from Tunnel Vision to Funnel Vision   97

Cultivating the Act of Witnessing Awareness   99

Exercise: Internal-Dialogue Assessment   101

Meditation: Anyone Can Do It   102

Thinking Thousands of Thoughts a Day   103

Do Nothing or Do Everything?   105

Wondering How It Works   106

Living a Spiritual Life   107

Checklist for Health: Spiritual Healing   112

CHAPTER 5. Emotional Health   113

Do You Run Your Emotions, or Do Your Emotions Run You?   115

Tools for Establishing a Healthy Emotional Life   116

Emotional Clearing for Each Dosha   123

Exercise: Your Emotional Healing Plan   127
Checklist for Health: Emotional Healing   130

CHAPTER 6. Healing Your Past   **131**

What Is Your Story?   131
Exercise: The Stories from Your Past   133
Exercise: Your New Reality   134
Understanding Why You Have a Past   134
Finding the Lesson and Moving On   137
The Seven Main Chakras: Opening Blocked Energy   139
Let Go of Your Past by Taking Three Lessons to the Future   148
Exercise: Your Three Lessons to Take to Your Fulfilling Future   148
Checklist for Health: Healing Your Past   149

CHAPTER 7. Relationship Health   **151**

We Are Social Beings Meant to Be in Relationships with Others   154
Life Is Not Balanced without Healthy and Loving Relationships   155
Twelve Traits of Healthy Relationships   159
*Exercise: Taking Inventory of Your Relationship
    Using the Twelve Traits*   166
Communicating Compassionately   170
Minding the Doshas in Relationships   173
Creating the Relationships You Desire   176
Steps to Attract the Right Mate   178
Checklist for Health: Healing Your Relationships   180

CHAPTER 8. Occupational Health   **183**

The Daily Grind   184
Doing What You Love and Loving What You Do   184
Discovering the Higher Purpose of Having a Career   185
Finding Dharma in a Career That Is Not Exactly Your Dharma   188
Honoring Your True Nature: Ideal Work for Vata, Pitta, Kapha   189
*Exercise: Creating a Plan for Transforming Your Current Job
    or Finding Your Ideal Job*   192
Checklist for Health: A Healthy Occupation   193

CHAPTER 9. Financial Health   195

   Your Financial Situation and Your Health   196
   Getting Rid of a Poverty Mind-Set   197
   Exercise: Taking Stock of Your Beliefs about Money   198
   Honoring Money as Energy: Giving to Receive   199
   Exercise: A Commitment to Financial Giving   201
   Your Plan to Abolish Debt and Create Wealth in Your Life   202
   Checklist for Health: Healing Your Finances   206

CHAPTER 10. Environmental Health   207

   Maximizing Healthy Sensory Input   209
   Outlining the Environments in My Daily Life   215
   Exercise: Space-Clearing Commitment   216
   The Dosha Response to Environment   217
   Reconnecting to the Outer Environment:
      Living outside Our Boxes   219
   Exercise: Ways You Can Live Outside Your Boxes   221
   Checklist for Health: Healing Your Environments   222

CHAPTER 11. Breaking a Spoke of the Wheel   223

   Dealing with Illness While Learning an Ayurvedic Lifestyle   224
   Healing from Addictions   226
   What If You Get Stuck on One Spoke and Cannot Move On?   227

CHAPTER 12. Rolling Smoothly: Enjoying the Ride   229

   Karmic Action: Doing What's Right   229
   On Being Gentle, Humble, Loving, and Kind   231

APPENDIX: Sun Salutations (Surya Namaskar)   233

NOTES   241

GLOSSARY OF SANSKRIT TERMS   243

RECOMMENDED WEBSITES AND AYURVEDIC RESOURCES   247

REFERENCES AND RECOMMENDED READING   249

INDEX   251

ABOUT THE AUTHOR   265

FOREWORD

The moment you are old enough to take the wheel,
responsibility lies with you.

— J. K. ROWLING

The quest for better health and energy is at the forefront
of many Americans' minds nowadays. According to the CDC,
the leading cause of death and disability in the United States
today is chronic diseases. Heart disease and cancer top the list
in claiming lives, and arthritis, diabetes, and obesity are their
cohorts in rendering millions of Americans disabled.

About half of all adults in the U.S. suffer from one or more
of the above-named chronic diseases. Are you one of them?
Do you want to avoid being included in these unfortunate statistics?

If you've picked up this book because you've heard about
Ayurveda or Ayurvedic medicine and wondered what it is, how
it works, and if it could help you, you're ready to get in the

driver's seat for a ride that will transform and improve your health and life. In *The Wheel of Healing with Ayurveda* Michelle Fondin makes the esoteric and ancient science of Ayurveda accessible to all readers who simply have a desire to improve their health. Her book will introduce you to Ayurveda and supply you with simple, practical, and creative ways to improve every aspect of your health.

My husband, Ayurvedic doctor and educator Dr. Shekhar Annambhotla, has witnessed the transformation of clients' health through their conscious shift to an Ayurvedic lifestyle. At his Ojas Ayurveda Wellness Center in our hometown of Coopersburg, Pennsylvania, he has helped clients suffering from obesity, arthritis, cancer, depression, constipation, insomnia, asthma, and other chronic conditions to incorporate principles of Ayurveda into their lives and make major improvements in their overall health. His compassionate and holistic approach inspired one client struggling with obesity to begin sipping hot water throughout the day, switch her main meal from dinner to lunch, and reduce her consumption of heavy sweets and meats. These simple changes added up to a tremendous amount of weight loss, a huge gain in energy and vitality, and improvements in other areas of her life. "The wheel" was truly set in motion.

Another client who had suffered with insomnia for over ten years was beginning to feel its debilitating effects as it led to more serious health problems. She had tried a variety of prescription sleep medications with poor results due to the side effects she experienced. As with many of my husband's first-time clients, she was at a point where she was compelled to take her health into her own hands. When she and Dr. Shekhar sat down to consider her diet, daily habits, and lifestyle, he gave her a few tips that she could easily follow to start getting the sleep she so desperately needed. Within a *couple of days* of doing a daily oil massage for herself before her shower, eliminating coffee, drinking a cup of warm milk with some tasty Ayurvedic herbs mixed in an hour before bedtime, and massaging the soles of her feet with warm oil at night, she was sleeping through the night regularly without any drugs or medications. She followed this up at Ojas Ayurveda Wellness Center with a series of gentle detoxification therapies (*panchakarma*), which helped correct deep-rooted imbalances in her physiology.

These examples of dramatic improvements in health as a result of making simple changes are exactly what Ayurveda is all about. Ayurveda shines even brighter when used to maintain good health and prevent diseases from taking root in our bodies. When I met my husband, I had long been interested in healthy eating, yoga, meditation, and holistic health approaches. I was intrigued by the ageless knowledge of Ayurveda and interested to know more about how it could improve my health. I ended up falling in love with both my husband and Ayurveda. His commitment, passion, and energy to share the wisdom of Ayurveda have been keeping our family, and the lives of everyone he touches, healthy and vibrant.

Association of Ayurvedic Professionals of North America (AAPNA), founded by Dr. Shekhar in 2002, has been offering free bimonthly educational phone conference calls for all since 2008. Each call features a speaker from the community of Ayurveda, yoga, and integrative medicine. When Michelle Fondin presented *The Wheel of Healing with Ayurveda* in September 2014, my husband knew that this was a book that would benefit anyone who was ready to make a positive change in their health.

Just as Patanjali, the father of yoga, defined eight limbs, or paths, of yoga, Michelle Fondin identifies and explains eight spokes in the wheel of health. She names these eight vital areas of life as dharma, or purpose in life; physical health; emotional health, including relationships and healing your past; spiritual health; environmental health; occupational health; and financial health. And at the center of this wheel of eight spokes is you. Fondin equips you with all you need to begin taking responsibility for your health using Ayurvedic principles. She includes a dosha assessment questionnaire to help you determine your individual mind-body type (*prakruti*), asks questions to help you discover your dharma, offers creative ideas for making your dharma a reality, provides tips on creating a personalized Ayurvedic eating plan, outlines an emotional healing plan, and presents many other essential lists, plans, and checklists. Work through this book from beginning to end making use of these resources, and you will achieve what you seek — yourself steadily driving forward on the path of health and wellness.

— Sudha Bulusu and Dr. Shekhar Annambhotla,
founder of Ojas Ayurveda Wellness Center and
Association of Ayurvedic Professionals of North America
(AAPNA)

ACKNOWLEDGMENTS

Thank you to Marina, Mathieu, and Xavier: You three are the lights of my life, who have helped me through the darkness and continue to light the path. With all my love, Mom.

To Amy Piper for modeling for the sun salutation photos: thank you, Amy!

Thank you to the staff at the Ayurvedic Path, who continue to give extraordinary service to our members at the studio.

And thanks to my Ayurvedic clients, who taught me what it's like to serve you and guide you to greater health.

To my mom: you were the first person to show me how to use inspiration and visualization posted on the bathroom mirror. Thank you for all those prayers and inspirational quotes.

To my love, Eric: thank you for being love.

MY STORY

Looking back to my earliest memory of health, I know I have always been health conscious but not necessarily healthy. At age twelve, I read Richard Simmons's book on weight loss and watched his videos. I went on to practice Jane Fonda–style workouts and started taking yoga at age eighteen. And so my passion for healthy living began.

But it wasn't until I was twenty-eight years old and the mother of two small children that my life took a sharp turn. I received the devastating news that no one ever wants to hear: "You have cancer." My diagnosis was thyroid cancer. All through the process, I kept asking the doctors, "What caused me to get cancer?" None of them could give me a remotely intelligible answer. I was dissatisfied with this lack of knowledge. Deep within me, I knew there had to be a reason why, at twenty-eight, I had allowed myself to become ill. And I didn't stop until I found that reason.

In a serendipitous event, I was led to Ayurveda, a five-thousand-year-old medical system developed in India. A friend handed me the book *Perfect Health*, by Dr. Deepak Chopra, and it introduced me to a medical system that understood my question. The practice of Ayurveda takes you to the root cause of illness by helping you understand how it originates in you.

After some time, I began practicing an Ayurvedic lifestyle and saw results. I did not refuse traditional allopathic treatment, however, and went through two surgeries and radioactive iodine treatments. But Ayurveda helped me on my path to healing, because at my core I knew that if I didn't discover the "why," I would only allow myself to get sick again. I also combed through every aspect of my life to search for answers. My logic was that, even if one area of my life stayed out of balance, I was opening myself up to illness. The idea for this book came out of my multifaceted approach to healing. My journey through illness and into wellness again made me believe that if I was frustrated by the current medical system, with its lack of answers, there must be countless others who are equally frustrated.

The Wheel of Healing with Ayurveda is designed to help you find the answers you seek by discovering your own inner healer. The advice I offer you is practical, easy, logical, and intuitive. Ayurveda takes a balanced approach and does not suggest you go to extremes. Be wary of any health plan that does. Know that, like anything authentic, change takes time. Be patient with yourself and don't expect results overnight. On my personal journey, it was three years after my cancer treatment before I felt I was in optimal health. That's longer than most people will take. But if I had given up, I wouldn't be where I am today, at age forty-three: much healthier than I ever was before age twenty-eight.

To quote one of my favorite teachers, Dr. Chopra: "Ayurveda is not about adding years to your life, it's about adding life to your years." Let's begin adding life to your years. You came to your life, this parenthesis in time, so you could live it.

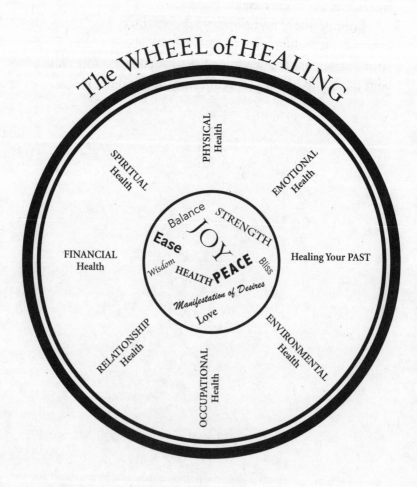

REINVENTING *the* WHEEL?

In the current economic, political, and social climate in the United States, the topic of health is more important than ever. At the time of this writing, in 2014, a major part of the American population is obese. According to the most recent figures released by the Centers for Disease Control and Prevention, 35.7 percent of people in this country are overweight.[1] Seven out of ten deaths among Americans each year result from chronic diseases. Heart disease, cancer, and stroke account for more than 50 percent of all deaths each year.[2] And the following statistic is staggering: in 2005, 133 million Americans, or one out of every two adults (50 percent), had a least one chronic illness.[3] And what do all these illnesses have in common? All are almost 100 percent preventable.

Yet the problem of illness continues. Health care costs have become astronomical; and even with our government-sponsored health care, costs will continue to rise. We have developed innovative technology, great resources for research, and experimental medicines, all in an effort to cure any illness known to humankind. Still we continue to become more ill as a whole as the years pass. What are the reasons for this incongruence?

One reason may be the discovery of disease in its later stages. Many people have a heart attack or stroke, or learn they have cancer, when their disease is well advanced. In those cases, all the technology or medicine in the world may not help them, so they may simply remain ill. A second reason may be the fragile state of many patients. Elderly individuals and small children are more susceptible to certain illnesses, and the medicines or procedures used to treat them may cause their bodies more harm than good.

Cost is another reason many people remain ill. Up until January 2014, many Americans had no health insurance, or they had poor health insurance. In either case, a sick person was more likely to wait until the symptoms were unbearable before going to the doctor. And even then, many treatments were cost prohibitive and patients literally could not access them.

One of the most common reasons for illness today is lifestyle. What we do, and what we don't do, is killing us. This news is actually more good than bad, though. For the most part, we are in direct control of our lifestyle. Even if we're skeptical, we can, by changing certain daily routines and habits, improve our health.

At some point in time, responsibility for our wellness shifted to someone *out there*. Somehow, we relinquished control of our health to someone or something else: doctors, health insurance companies, drug companies, food growers, chemists, and, yes, even advertisers. This relinquishment has spiraled so far out of control that we no longer know who to blame for our ill health. The solution doesn't appear to lie in the future, so let's turn backward, to the wisdom of the ages.

The concept discussed in *The Wheel of Healing* brings control and responsibility back to you. By taking charge of your life and learning how to use the eight "spokes" of the Ayurvedic wheel of healing, you can work your way toward wellness. Taking charge does not, however, necessarily mean that your health will always be perfect. There are too many variables to permit predicting such an outcome. But rest assured that by making changes you will be better equipped to process illness when and if it occurs.

As you regain control, any fear you have about your health will dissipate. As your fear dissipates, you will be able to focus your energy on living life to the fullest. Living your life to the fullest will enable you to live the life you aspire to. As you refocus, you will learn to expand your definition of health. For the most part, when we think of health we refer to our physical body. If our body is strong and pain free, we declare that we are healthy. But if our body is experiencing aches and pains or other indications of illness, we claim we are sick. The shift that is about to take place in your belief system will result from embracing the healing system that I discuss in this book.

Throughout the book, I refer to Ayurveda, a mind-body medical system from India. My training in and practice of Ayurveda has allowed me to utilize its concept of wholeness in my life and the lives of hundreds of clients, who notice immediate results when applying its principles.

The principle of wholeness may be understood from the following example. Suppose you are in the market to buy a new home. You've decided on several different qualities that you look for in a home — for example, you spend a lot of time in the kitchen cooking gourmet meals, and so a beautiful, useful kitchen is your number one priority. But you would also like a home with large windows, a decent-sized master bath, and four bedrooms, and it must be reasonably priced and located on a quiet street. Once you find a real estate agent, you explain your passion for cooking and how you enjoy coming home from work, preparing meals, and eating with your family. You then explain the other things you'd like in a home. The well-intentioned agent, however, hears only the part about the kitchen and proceeds to show you a series of homes with terrific kitchens, paying no attention to your other specifications. After viewing homes with beautiful kitchens and high price tags, cramped master baths, and small windows — homes that are all located in the middle of the city or have only two bedrooms — you complain to the agent that he's not showing you what you want. He responds, "But you said you love to cook in a well-equipped kitchen. All these homes have fantastic kitchens."

Seeing health as related only to the physical body is the same as buying a house because of a single room. Most of us would agree that it takes many different aspects to compel us to purchase a home. A home is a big investment of our resources and time. If we base the purchase on one aspect, we may find ourselves with big problems later on when we discover faulty plumbing, a tattered roof, or restricted closet space. Like our home, our health is a big investment. Learning how to live life according to a holistic model requires an investment of our time and money. But if we adopt the principles that I outline in the following chapters, the payoff will immeasurably outweigh the cost.

But it's also true that, without good physical health, we may find it difficult to focus on the many aspects of the wheel that I introduce here. For that reason we will begin our journey with dharma, meaning "purpose in life," and with physical health and its close companion, emotional health. Relationship health and healing your past are subdivisions of emotional health, and we will address those as well. The next aspect, spiritual health, ties physical and emotional health together. We will then delve into three other aspects of health: environmental health, occupational health, and financial health.

Why the Wheel?

I chose the analogy of the wheel for many reasons. First, a wheel is a continuum: it has no beginning and no end. The integrity of the wheel is extremely important, as in the case of a bicycle wheel. If you don't know how to ride a bike, it may be impossible to imagine that it will support your weight and move forward on two skinny wheels. Yet it works. But if a wheel is missing some spokes, or the rim is bent, balancing becomes more difficult. If you continue to ride a bike that is missing spokes, it may support your weight for a time; but the wheel will eventually collapse from the lack of wholeness. So too with our bodies and our health. We may get by, for a time, without elements essential to our health — for example, we may exercise too little or omit vegetables from our diet. But if we continue, eventually our health will fail. It is inevitable. The mystery in human health is multifaceted. We cannot attain perfect health simply by eating properly while ignoring exercise or emotional health. To observe this point, talk to someone who eats healthfully but doesn't have loving relationships. Or talk to someone who exercises daily but hates his job. Once you do this, the concept of wholeness will begin to be revealed to you.

The second reason I chose the wheel is because you can touch it on any side. You don't have to pass through a maze to access a certain area. You don't have to complete your work on one side in order to start another. You can start on one side, then turn the wheel around and begin on the opposite side. As you will see, all parts are completely integrated. And when you begin an exploration of one side, you immediately begin to access other sides without consciously starting. Perhaps a lack in one area of your life led you to pick up this book. If that's the case, you can begin with that particular area of the wheel and move on to the next.

Taking Back Your Health and Your Life

You need not go far to get advice on how you should live your life or improve your health. We are bombarded today, more than ever, with the latest and greatest trend. From pomegranate seeds and goji berries to chia seeds, every week it's something different, an additional thing that may take a place on our already crammed lists. If it's not the latest food or supplement, it's the next powerful drug claiming to make us younger and happier or to give us a better sex life. All this advice, whether good or bad, always does one specific thing: it draws us outside ourselves to seek wellness; and in the end, this makes us crazy. Because, to be honest, who do you listen to? Really, *who* can you trust when the advice is changing so rapidly? At the time of this writing, many of my clients are turning to daytime talk shows for advice on diet, exercise, and balancing their lives. Frankly, I have nothing against talk shows, and I'm sure that guests on the shows have plenty of knowledge. But again, much of the advice doesn't empower the spectators to take charge of their own health by tuning in to what's going on inside. And since much of the information is piecemeal, it doesn't necessarily give them the tools to follow a complete program to get and stay healthy.

Ayurvedic medicine teaches people to first look inward. Get to know yourself inside and out. Know what makes you tick. And what makes you tick is probably different from what makes the other people in your life tick. If you do not take this crucial step first, no sprout, herb, vitamin, juice, or drug will help you.

Back in the 1980s, the rising trend was to see fat in the diet as a bad thing. Everything had to be fat-free or you could not lose weight, according to the claims. As a result, the food companies began producing fat-free everything — even fat-free butter, which is naturally 100 percent fat. I was eighteen years old at the height of this trend and, like many teenage girls, wanted to lose a few pounds. So I began a fat-free diet. I made sure not to add any fat whatsoever to my diet.

Then a couple of things happened. First, I began to lose my appetite. Food literally made me sick. I could not stomach fat-free cheese, yogurt, or dressings. I found them too sweet and sickening. Second, I began to experience headaches and a slump in energy, and my mood was terrible. I did manage to lose some weight, but at the cost of my well-being. Finally, after a few months, as happens with any diet that excludes a major food group, my body retaliated. I gave up, pigged out on all the fat my body had been craving, and regained the weight. Years later, when I discovered Ayurvedic medicine, I learned why my body had responded so poorly to the fat-free diet. First of all, our bodies need fat to survive. This is especially true of the human brain, which is 60 percent fat, making it the fattiest organ in the body. Moreover, my Ayurvedic mind-body type is composed of generous amounts of space and air. The absence of fat only increases these elements in the body-mind, and for me this led to disaster.

What often happens is that our body gives us signals of discomfort when we do something that is not nourishing us. Then our mind overrides those signals with reasons why this thing is, in fact, good for us. Even when in reality it's not. At those moments we are overriding our body's natural intelligence.

Taking Responsibility for Your Health

One concept you must embrace before beginning this journey is the concept of taking responsibility for your own health and well-being. By purchasing this book you've taken the first step. But fully knowing that you are the one directly influencing your health is the key to turning your health around for the better.

The shift that you will make is from a victim mind-set to a responsibility-based mind-set. One is reactive, and the other is proactive. If you are to heal completely and live more fully, it's essential that you let go of the victim mind-set. That mind-set says, "I can't get healthy because…" or "I'm unhealthy because…my husband [or my wife, my job, my mother, and so on] stresses me out." When we have that mind-set, we get angry when the people around us don't respond favorably when we are ill. My question to you is: How can you expect others to care more about your health than you do?

Taking responsibility for your health doesn't mean blaming yourself. It simply means taking charge. Don't wait for your spouse to cook you healthy meals; instead, go shopping, use the principles in this book, and make dinner yourself. If you don't know how to cook, take a cooking class. And don't put off exercise by waiting for that next paycheck to come so you can join a gym. Put on a pair of sneakers and comfortable clothing now, get outside, and walk for twenty or thirty minutes. There will always be excuses that let you avoid improving your health, more excuses than you can probably conjure up in your mind right now. But there is an equal number of opportunities to grasp each and every day. When you make this shift, you can be a beacon of light for others to follow.

Focus on why you desire health. Let that desire be your guide and motivation. And then go for it. You are the one who cares the most about you. And finally, know that this is a journey. It may commence here, but it's a journey that will last your lifetime. So let the journey begin!

Exercise: Your Commitment to Yourself

Here or in your journal, write down the commitment you are making to yourself by reading this book. Then sign and date the page, following the example below.

My commitment to myself during the process of reading *The Wheel of Healing*:

Signature: _____

Date: _____

CHAPTER ONE

A QUICK IMMERSION *in* AYURVEDA

Even if a physician has profound book knowledge, without entering into the patient's heart with the flame of love and the light of knowledge, one cannot properly treat disease.

— CHARAKA SAMHITA (SACRED AYURVEDIC TEXT)

Ayurveda is a vast body of knowledge. Some have even said this knowledge is as vast as the ocean, and that it's difficult for a practitioner to master it completely. Let's start with the basics that you will need to know to begin easily living an Ayurvedic lifestyle.

What Is Ayurveda?

Ayurveda is mind-body medicine that originated in India at least five thousand years ago. The name *Ayurveda* comes from two Sanskrit (an ancient language of India) words: *ayus*, meaning "life," and *veda*, which means "science" or "knowledge." So the name literally means the "science of life." Ayurveda is a complete medical system or science that includes observation; diagnosis, treatment, and prevention of disease; detoxification and rejuvenation of the body; surgery; and herbal medicine. Ayurveda is called a consciousness-based system of medicine because the practitioner seeks to understand the patient fully before recommending or administering treatment, and because the practitioner works not only on observation but also on intuition. The Ayurvedic practitioner knows that the patient is not simply flesh and bones but a dynamic being with a mind, a body, emotions, a soul, and a spirit. As the Charaka Samhita states, the physician needs to enter the heart of the patient "with the flame of love." If she does not, she cannot help him. I believe this statement points to what has been lost in allopathic, or Western, medicine, and to what can be found in Ayurvedic medicine.

Why Ayurveda Rather Than Another Healing Modality?

Ayurveda is all-encompassing. The practice of Ayurveda addresses diet, lifestyle, seasonal and daily routines, herbal medicine, massage or touch therapy, detoxification of the body, energy work, spiritual practice through yoga and meditation, and surgery. The philosophy behind Ayurveda says that if it works, then you should try it. Even if you apply the principles in this guide, you can still continue to follow your physician's protocol, take prescribed medications, and make use of other methods used in allopathic medicine.

Another reason to follow an Ayurvedic practice is that it's the most complete medical system on the planet. Other disciplines of Ayurveda, which I don't have space to examine here, include Ayurvedic astrology and the study of object placement and space.

Finally, Ayurveda focuses on the practice of preventive

medicine first. Awareness of the body, mind, and intellect can lead you to recognize subtle changes that occur before full-blown illness erupts. Reversing subtle changes in the body is much easier than curing a disease. By learning little things and applying them, you can make a big difference in your health.

Balance versus Imbalance

One major difference between Western medicine and Ayurveda is that Ayurveda looks at health and illness as a matter of balance and imbalance. If a person is balanced, she is healthy, vibrant, energetic, alive, happy, and motivated, and her skin and eyes glow. When a person is out of balance, she is dull, achy, tired, lethargic, worried, nervous, or depressed. Whether or not physical symptoms are present, Ayurveda can detect that a person is out of balance, and this imbalance will ultimately lead to a manifestation of symptoms and disease if not corrected. Discovering this imbalance before the patient becomes ill gives the Ayurvedic practitioner a little more wiggle room to help the patient. Patients go to the doctor because they are uncomfortable. And if the doctor doesn't detect any physical symptoms or abnormalities, then all too often he sends the patient home in exactly the condition he arrived in. But the Ayurvedic practitioner, through observation, palpation, and a series of questions, can easily detect the state of imbalance and help tweak the patient's health back into balance by recommending alterations in diet, exercise, yoga, meditation, and lifestyle, along with emotional clearing or herbs.

The Ayurvedic Definition of Health

Often, clients come to me for Ayurvedic consultations who claim to be completely healthy. On the questionnaires I send them before the first visit, they write, under the inquiries about their physical health and emotional health, that they are in "excellent" or "very good" shape. These same clients may be notably overweight or addicted to alcohol, or they may struggle with insomnia or anxiety or some other complaint that prevents them from living their lives to the fullest. Upon further questioning, they admit, "Yes, I have a few pounds to lose." Or: "I can't end my day without a drink." Or: "I haven't slept more than five hours a night in ten years."

The shift I will ask you to make in your definition of health is from one that is typical of a Western mind-set — "If I have no symptoms, I am healthy" — to an Ayurvedic definition: "Health is an integration of my mind, emotions, soul, spirit, physical body, and purpose in life." If one of these is out of balance, they are all out of balance, rest assured. In the following chapters, you will learn to recognize when you are out of balance and will discover that you possess the tools to regain true health.

The Mahabhutas: The Great Elements

When Ayurveda was in its infancy, sages called *rishis*, or seers, observed people and nature. What they noticed was that people reacted differently to similar stimuli. For example, if you walk into a room with a friend, you may find yourself freezing while your friend complains that it's too warm. Or if you and your spouse walk outside into the bright sunlight, he or she may need to immediately put on sunglasses to appreciate the outdoors, while you enjoy allowing the sun to penetrate your face. These differences, the rishis realized, occurred because each person has a unique dynamic, a different mind-body type based on the five elements that exist everywhere. Those five elements are space (*akasha*), air (*vayu*), fire (*tejas*), water (*jala*), and earth (*prithivi*). In Sanskrit, these elements are called the *mahabhutas*, or "great elements," and they influence all other elements. The five elements make up the three principal *doshas*, or mind-body types, in Ayurveda.

An Introduction to the Doshas

The three principal doshas, or mind-body types, are Vata, Pitta, and Kapha. The Vata principle (pronounced VAH-ta) is composed of the elements space and air. "Space" means the vast open space, or ether, but also the space in a room, the space in a box, or the space between your cells. In order for air to move and circulate, it needs space. So these two elements work harmoniously together. The Pitta principle (pronounced PIT-ta) is composed of the elements fire and water, which together have transformational qualities. And the Kapha principle (pronounced KAF-fa) is composed of water and earth. These elements exist everywhere on our planet and in the universe, in different quantities. Since we are part of the planet and universe, the elements exist within each of us too.

Each person has all three doshas in his or her mind-body constitution. But the proportion of these doshas is different in everyone. General trends in doshic makeup usually exist in families, since genes are shared. But sometimes that's not the case, since environment, geographical location, date, time, and season of birth often influence a person's *prakruti*, or true nature.

To determine your prakruti, please take the following Mind-Body Type Test. When you assess each of the statements, think about how you've acted, reacted, or been for your whole life. If a statement has been true some of the time or during

certain periods of your life, decide how accurately it describes
you on average. The test will yield accurate information only
if you are truthful to yourself. The results will guide you as
you improve your health and come back to what is a naturally
balanced state for you.

The Ayurvedic Mind-Body Type Test

Please assess each of the following statements as it applies
to you, on average, for your whole life. If a statement
doesn't apply to you at all, score it a 0. If it is absolutely
you, score it a 5. Score a statement 1 or 2 if it describes
you rarely; give it a 3 if it applies some of the time; and
score it a 4 if it applies most of the time.

SECTION I

1. I have always had a thin physique. I don't gain weight easily.	0	1	2	3	4	5
2. I walk quickly. I'm always at the head of the pack.	0	1	2	3	4	5
3. I get nervous or anxious easily.	0	1	2	3	4	5
4. I eat quickly and my family says I should slow down.	0	1	2	3	4	5
5. My mind is very creative.	0	1	2	3	4	5
6. I learn things quickly, but I also forget quickly.	0	1	2	3	4	5
7. I like to pace when I talk on the phone.	0	1	2	3	4	5

8. When I was a kid, people said I fidgeted a lot.	0	1	2	3	4	5
9. Constipation is often an issue for me.	0	1	2	3	4	5
10. My mind is very active and sometimes restless.	0	1	2	3	4	5
11. When there is a conflict, I ask myself, "What did I do wrong?"	0	1	2	3	4	5
12. Left on my own, I would eat and sleep at different times each day.	0	1	2	3	4	5
13. I get bored easily if I'm not constantly on the move.	0	1	2	3	4	5
14. When I go into a room, I often feel that it's too cold.	0	1	2	3	4	5
15. I often have dry, rough skin.	0	1	2	3	4	5
16. Weather that is cold and windy bothers me more than most people.	0	1	2	3	4	5
17. Sometimes people accuse me of being "airheaded."	0	1	2	3	4	5
18. My friends say that I'm talkative.	0	1	2	3	4	5
19. I'm a light sleeper; I have difficulty getting to sleep or I sleep restlessly.	0	1	2	3	4	5
20. I like to start new projects, activities, or hobbies but have a hard time sticking with them.	0	1	2	3	4	5

TOTAL SCORE FOR SECTION I: _____

SECTION II

1. My eyes are sensitive to the sun.	0	1	2	3	4	5
2. I have a medium build.	0	1	2	3	4	5
3. My appetite is strong. If I want, I can eat a large quantity.	0	1	2	3	4	5
4. I don't like to have my time wasted.	0	1	2	3	4	5
5. I have a strong desire to learn new things.	0	1	2	3	4	5
6. My days are typically planned. I like to follow an agenda.	0	1	2	3	4	5
7. When I overeat or am upset, I tend to get acid reflux, heartburn, or a burning sensation in my stomach.	0	1	2	3	4	5
8. Many people consider me stubborn.	0	1	2	3	4	5
9. In my actions I'm precise and orderly.	0	1	2	3	4	5
10. I like to see things in their place.	0	1	2	3	4	5
11. When there is a conflict, I wonder why people can't see things the way I do.	0	1	2	3	4	5
12. If I don't eat my meals on time, I get cranky and irritable.	0	1	2	3	4	5
13. I enjoy spending time outdoors. It exhilarates me.	0	1	2	3	4	5
14. I often feel that a room is too warm.	0	1	2	3	4	5

	0	1	2	3	4	5
15. I have a tendency to break out in acne, hives, and rashes, or I have skin redness.	0	1	2	3	4	5
16. It's common for me to have loose stools or to have a bowel movement more than twice a day.	0	1	2	3	4	5
17. I am quick to anger, but I quickly forget about it.	0	1	2	3	4	5
18. My friends say I'm intense.	0	1	2	3	4	5
19. Spicy food aggravates my stomach.	0	1	2	3	4	5
20. When I want something, I'm very determined in my efforts to get it.	0	1	2	3	4	5

TOTAL SCORE FOR SECTION II: _____

SECTION III

	0	1	2	3	4	5
1. People say I'm "big boned."	0	1	2	3	4	5
2. I walk slowly. I don't understand why people have to hurry all the time.	0	1	2	3	4	5
3. If I have a lot of stress in my life, I don't want to deal with it.	0	1	2	3	4	5
4. I eat slowly. I'm the last one to finish at the table.	0	1	2	3	4	5
5. It takes me longer than others to learn things, but I never forget what I've learned.	0	1	2	3	4	5
6. I can just look at a piece of cake and gain ten pounds.	0	1	2	3	4	5

7. I like to snuggle up on the couch with a good book and stay for hours without moving.	0	1	2	3	4	5
8. I like to sleep, especially in the morning. I don't consider myself a morning person.	0	1	2	3	4	5
9. My digestion is slow. I feel heavy after meals.	0	1	2	3	4	5
10. I would rather watch sports on TV than participate in athletic activity.	0	1	2	3	4	5
11. When there is a conflict, I want to crawl into my bed and forget it happened.	0	1	2	3	4	5
12. I don't understand people who say they're not hungry. If there's food in front of me, I want to eat it.	0	1	2	3	4	5
13. I need at least eight hours of sleep to feel comfortable the next day.	0	1	2	3	4	5
14. Weather that is cool and damp bothers me.	0	1	2	3	4	5
15. I think I'm affected by seasonal affective disorder (SAD).	0	1	2	3	4	5
16. I don't like change very much. I enjoy things staying the same.	0	1	2	3	4	5
17. My friends and family say I'm affectionate and a good listener.	0	1	2	3	4	5
18. I have problems with mucus, excess phlegm, or chronic sinus problems and allergies.	0	1	2	3	4	5

| 19. I have had a weight problem most of my life. | 0 | 1 | 2 | 3 | 4 | 5 |
| 20. I am slow and methodical in all my actions. | 0 | 1 | 2 | 3 | 4 | 5 |

TOTAL SCORE FOR SECTION III: _____

Total Scores and the Doshas

Transfer the total scores for each section to the blanks shown below. Then determine which of the three is your highest score, and check the list of possible mind-body types to find the corresponding dosha. If your highest score is more than 85 points, it's likely that you're a single dosha type. If your second score is close to your first score and at least 10 points above your third, you are a two-dosha type. For example, if you scored 73 points for section I, 54 points for section II, and 27 points for section III, you would be a Vata-Pitta. Only in very rare instances is someone tridoshic — that is, characterized by a mind-body type composed of equal amounts of all three doshas.

Section I score: _____ Vata
Section II score: _____ Pitta
Section III score: _____ Kapha

The possible mind-body types:
Vata   Pitta-Vata
Pitta   Pitta-Kapha
Kapha   Kapha-Vata
Vata-Pitta   Kapha-Pitta
Vata-Kapha

The purpose of the Mind-Body Type Test is to identify your natural state of being, not to make sure all three doshas are equally strong in you or to choose the traits you think you might like. When a person is in balance, he or she possesses all the positive traits of all the doshas. For example, a Kapha type is naturally trustworthy and faithful. That does not mean a Pitta or a Vata person cannot have those traits too. It simply means that trustworthiness and faithfulness come easily for a Kapha type, and that when in balance, Pitta and Vata types also tend to be aligned with these positive traits. However, when a person is out of balance, he or she usually shows the negative traits of the dominant dosha first; if the condition continues, negative traits of the other doshas appear, too. To return to my example of the Kapha person (who is naturally trustworthy and faithful), a negative outcome for an imbalanced Kapha is possessiveness and greed. And if the imbalance continues, the possessiveness can also lead to anger, which is a normal Pitta imbalance, or to anxiety, which is a normal Vata imbalance.

Once you determine your mind-body type, or prakruti, read the description of each dosha. Keep in mind that each description represents a classic example of that mind-body type and may apply to you only in part. It's common to see several traits of your dominant dosha in yourself, a few traits of your secondary dosha, and maybe one or two traits of the dosha for which you scored the least number of points.

Vata Dosha: The Wind Principle

Possessing a dosha composed of space and air, the Vata person is thin and light and has angular features. Imagine the qualities of space: vast, open, infinite, and cold; and the qualities of air: moving, cool, changing, unpredictable, rough, drying. A Vata type has these qualities in his body and mind. Vatas are quick.

They move fast, talk fast, walk fast. They think and learn fast but also forget fast. Vatas are easily excitable, engaging in the latest activities, fads, or fashions. They are fun, creative, communicative, and enterprising. Like the wind, they stay for a time then move on to the next location. Being with a Vata type keeps you young and laughing, because they are playful, funny, and witty. But they can also be unpredictable and unreliable. Often they are accused of being "airheaded." Vatas resist routine, even though they need it, and forget to eat or sleep at times. It is typically Vata to start a project and not finish it, change jobs or relationships often, and spend money on trivialities.

When in balance, Vata types keep you on your toes with their boundless energy. But when out of balance, Vatas suffer from anxiety, panic attacks, weight loss, constipation, dry skin and eyes, aches and pains, and fear.

Pitta Dosha: The Fire Principle

Fire and water may seem like opposite qualities at first glance, but they work together to transform one thing into another. For example, if you make a batch of brownies, you mix together the dry ingredients and the wet ingredients. When you've finished stirring them together, you have a thick, wet, gloppy mixture. Factors that contribute to the wetness are generally eggs, water, and oil. Then you put the mixture in a pan and stick it in the oven to bake. Forty-five minutes later, you have brownies. But if you were to dig through the baked brownies to find the eggs, water, or oil, you would be unsuccessful. The reason is that the "fire," or the oven in this case, transformed the ingredients into something else. That's the transformative effect of Pitta.

Pitta types have a medium build. A Pitta has beautiful eyes with a penetrating gaze and a healthy glow to her skin. It is Pitta to want things to be in order, to be a perfectionist about details, and to not like having her time wasted. A Pitta is driven by education, learning new skills, gathering facts, and then sharing the knowledge with anyone who will listen. To others, Pittas are interesting, attractive, well spoken, and intense.

Physically, Pittas are like goats. They can eat anything they want, owing to a strong digestive fire, and will usually be fine. But they also tend to abuse their great digestion by overeating or eating too many spicy or fried foods, all of which aggravate Pitta.

When Pittas are in balance, they are strong leaders, passionate lovers, informative educators, and beautiful. But when a Pitta is out of balance, she spews fire, criticizing and judging everyone in her path. She's irritable, unpleasant, and furrows her brow a lot. She gets acid indigestion or irritable bowels and has a hard time digesting any type of food. Her skin gets red with anger and often breaks out.

Kapha Dosha: The Earth Principle

Composed of earth and water, which together create mud, Kapha is slow, wet, cold, thick, viscous, compact, and heavy. A Kapha type has a large build, big bones, and more fat under his skin than the other dosha types have. He has large, loving eyes and rosy cheeks. Kaphas move like the tortoise. They walk slowly, talk slowly, think and process things slowly, and don't worry much. It is Kapha to resist change, enjoy routine, and be methodical and affectionate. To others, Kaphas are grounding, steady, loving, and trustworthy, and they are great listeners. Kaphas have a difficult time understanding why they love food so much and gain weight easily. When in balance, Kaphas are the solid foundation of a family or company. Once a Kapha is out of balance, he gains weight, refuses to move off the couch, accumulates clutter, becomes possessive in relationships, and has excess mucus in his body. While all three mind-body types are at risk for depression when out of balance, a Kapha type is the quickest to become depressed, especially in late winter.

Interpreting Your Mind-Body Type

It's important that you understand a few facts about your mind-body type in order to help heal yourself. Different doshas respond to different treatments, and by knowing which dosha is out of balance or likely to be out of balance, you will know which direction to take. For example, if you've had chronic constipation for most of your life, or constipation becomes a problem during times of stress or travel, then pay attention to the Vata dosha to rebalance yourself. But if you have acid reflux as a result of overeating, eating while upset, or eating spicy food, you need to rebalance Pitta.

Since all three doshas exist in us, it's possible to experience an imbalance in any of the three. For example, suppose you have a Vata constitution and it's winter in Michigan. You've broken your leg, and you've been laid up on the couch for weeks. It's cold, you're upset that you can't move (Vata types are not well when they can't move), and you've been eating too much in an attempt to comfort yourself. Once you recover from the broken leg, you discover that you're tired most of the time, have a desire to sleep late in the morning, and have gained ten pounds. Because of the given situation, season, and circumstances, you, as a Vata, are now experiencing a Kapha imbalance. In this case, Kapha would be the appropriate dosha to rebalance.

Often in consultations I'm asked, "Can my doshas change throughout my life?" The answer is, your prakruti does not change, your *vikruti* changes. Your prakruti is the genetic hand you were dealt at the time of your conception. Just as you would have a difficult time permanently changing your eye color, you cannot change your prakruti. However, I have seen clients so terribly imbalanced that it appeared they had one prakruti, but after detailed questions, I discovered their true nature was totally different.

Vikruti is your current state. Most often, it's your state of imbalance. We are constantly swinging from balance to imbalance. If we live a healthy lifestyle according to our doshas and the Ayurvedic principles, we remain more or less balanced most of the time. However, if we continue to ignore our body's signs, eating whatever we feel like and living a sedentary or chemically abusive lifestyle, we will continue to pull ourselves out of balance. Disease doesn't happen overnight. We may think that it does, but subtle changes take place over days, months, years, and decades.

The question in your mind may now be: "Well, which dosha should I balance?" For the sake of simplicity, it's best to begin by balancing your dominant dosha, the dosha for which you scored the highest. Balancing a person's prakruti, especially when illness is present, can be a complicated matter, and it's best done under the guidance of an Ayurvedic practitioner. But I can assure you that if you apply the principles in this book, your health will improve exponentially. And once you're sold on the method, you can seek out an Ayurvedic practitioner in your area for more complicated health issues.

In *The Wheel of Healing*, I describe individual doshas as being aggravated and explain that they must be pacified. Pay attention to the six stages of disease, described in the following pages, in order to understand the concept of how disease develops. It may seem completely new and strange to you as a Western reader, but remember: this is wisdom of the ages.

This wisdom, passed on through generations and millennia, is sound. And once you understand how Ayurveda works, it will make complete sense.

The Six Stages of Disease

Stage 1. Accumulation

When focusing on your mind-body type, embrace this statement: You don't need more of what you already have. A Pitta has a fair amount of fire and water in his mind-body constitution. So by increasing the fire and water elements, you aggravate the Pitta dosha. *Accumulation* means that a dosha increases in an area of the body, usually an area where the dosha normally sits. For example, Vata is present in the colon. So when the air and space elements accumulate in the colon, it increases the amount in that area of the body. Since air and space are already fairly abundant in the colon, increased amounts can aggravate the colon.

Stage 2. Aggravation

The accumulation of the dosha begins to distort the normal function of the area it's occupying. In the colon example, a person with increased air and space elements may begin to experience bloating or abdominal discomfort but not really understand where it comes from.

Stage 3. Dissemination

The aggravated dosha begins to spread outside its normal zone. To continue our example, the person may begin to experience excess gas and have a feeling of general discomfort in the abdomen, decreased appetite, and fatigue.

Stage 4. Localization

The expanding dosha begins to settle in an area of the body that already has some weakness, such as a site of previous injury, a spot where a person has had surgery, or some other vulnerable place in the body. So now, the person with excess Vata that began in the colon may be experiencing gas and constipation but also upper back pain.

Stage 5. Manifestation

If the symptoms in stage 4 are ignored, they will be exacerbated and exaggerated in a given bodily space. For example, if the aggravated Vata moves up into the brain, the imbalance may manifest as a panic attack.

Stage 6. Disruption

At this stage, if the imbalance is not corrected, full-blown illness erupts. It could be a repeated acute attack (such as a panic attack, asthma attack, or heart attack), a chronic condition (lupus, fibromyalgia, heart disease), or a complete disruption of all the doshas, as is seen in cancer.

According to the Ayurvedic model, a Western doctor wouldn't be able to detect an abnormality until about the fourth or fifth stage. At this point, the seeds of illness have been planted and have been growing for some time. Often, a patient will go see a doctor in stage 3 or early stage 4 with complaints of fatigue, discomfort, and a general sense of "not feeling well." A Western physician will have a difficult time pinpointing the origin of the illness. She may ask a few questions and run some tests, and if all the tests come back "normal," she will write the complaint off as a virus or may even prescribe an antidepressant or another mood-lifting drug. Please don't get me wrong. I'm not blaming the medical community at all. Doctors have saved my life many times over. I was a very sick child and continued to be sick as a young adult. And it's because of Western medicine that I'm here today. But the model takes healing only to a certain level. Doctors simply don't have the tools to see the entire picture. However, this wasn't always the case.

Examples of physicians in the early twentieth century show that because of the intimate nature of villages and home life, physicians knew their patients personally. A doctor's personal relationship with not only the patient but also the patient's family, friends, and neighbors expanded his healing capability. Doctors in those days visited a sick patient's home. They observed the patient's environment and knew what else was happening in the patient's life. And since intimacy helps hone a person's intuitive skills, the doctors were also more intuitive. They didn't have the plethora of drugs available that we have today, so they had to rely a little more on common sense, compassion, observation, and relationship.

Let's fast-forward to today. Doctors are governed by health insurance companies, costly malpractice insurance, and the financial demands of big medical practices that they share with other doctors. All of them are under pressure to see an overlarge number of patients each day and don't have the luxury of getting to know their patients intimately. How can they become well acquainted with a patient in a fifteen-minute window of time or less? Moreover, in medical school, physicians are not taught compassion and given the tools for connection with a patient. Most take only one course in nutrition and lifestyle, and that may be optional. For the most part, they are taught pathology. They know how to diagnose and treat illness. Let me give you an example from my own experience.

After two surgeries for thyroid cancer, along with radioactive iodine therapy, I began feeling miserable. I was extremely fatigued, lacked motivation, was jittery, had brain fog, was fearful, and had panic attacks, to name a few symptoms. All of these can be signs of hypothyroidism. I went to my endocrinologist and explained the symptoms. He ran some tests and announced that all tests were normal and there was nothing wrong with me. After seeing the symptoms only increase, and after going through two more doctors who told me my symptoms were all in my head, I went to see Dr. Leonard Wisneski, an endocrinologist with a background in herbal medicine, acupuncture, and holistic healing. Dr. Wisneski walked into the examining room and opened his arms to give me a hug. After giving me a good squeeze, he tossed his file aside and asked, "So what's going on?" He listened intently while I poured my heart out to him, and then responded, "You're not crazy. You're going through post-traumatic stress disorder, and you're probably depleted nutritionally and on the wrong thyroid medication." Here's what he did right:

1. He addressed me as a human, and not simply as a patient, by hugging me.
2. He listened intently.
3. He believed what I was telling him.
4. He assured me that what I was telling him about my health was correct.
5. He told me there was a solution.
6. He offered a solution that was multifaceted and that addressed more than simply my symptoms.

As the quote from the Charaka Samhita says a physician must do, Dr. Wisneski entered the heart of his patient. In illness, there's a tremendous amount of fear. If through compassion, a physician can dispel the fear, symptoms improve.

But the physician must also have tools other than prescription medication and medical interventions.

An Ayurvedic doctor or practitioner can detect an illness at stage 1, well before symptoms appear. In an Ayurvedic consultation, a practitioner will make recommendations in order to balance doshas — through lifestyle, nutrition, meditation, and yoga and other forms of regular exercise. Preventive measures are recommended to stop the aggravation of a dosha, and this will arrest any symptoms.

Creating a Symptom Plan

The type of symptoms that may appear are specific to a certain mind-body type. For example, at some point in their lives Vata types will see symptoms of gas, bloating, constipation, nervousness, a racing mind, anxiety, panic attacks, loss of appetite, restless sleep, weight loss, and fear. Being Vata, it's inevitable. Healthy Vatas will see these symptoms less often, while unhealthy Vatas will see them more frequently.

Pitta types often see hyperacidity, acid reflux, diarrhea, acne, skin redness, hives, rashes, eye sensitivity, ulcers, canker sores, a ravenous appetite, nausea, anger, irritability, impatience, and self-criticism or criticism of others.

Kapha types usually experience lethargy, weight gain, inertia, hoarding, mild to moderate depression, laziness, water retention, sinusitis or allergy symptoms, asthma, and chronic bronchitis and wheezing.

Please take a few minutes to write down the symptoms that most often manifest in your life. If you're not certain, close your eyes and take a walk down memory lane to your earliest childhood memory, and then scan your lifetime. You will notice some patterns in yourself. Awareness of whether your typical symptoms are more typically Vata-, Pitta-, or Kapha-like will assist you in rebalancing yourself.

Exercise: Identifying Your Typical Symptoms

My typical symptoms throughout my life are:

Symptoms I've been experiencing in the past ninety days:

✔ Checklist for Health

An Introduction to Ayurveda

❏ Rate your physical and mental health today. Do you feel your health is poor, fair, good, very good, or excellent?

❏ Take the Mind-Body Type Test and determine your Ayurvedic mind-body type.

❏ Read the descriptions of the doshas and determine which one most resonates with who you are today.

❏ Create a list of your typical symptoms, including any that have occurred throughout your life.

CHAPTER TWO

The ENTIRE WHEEL

Living Your Dharma, or Life's Purpose

*Your purpose in life is to find your purpose
and give your whole heart and soul to it.*

— GAUTAMA BUDDHA

As a person who has read the first hundred pages of many
books and never gotten to the end, I'm starting with the most
important aspect of this program. If you get nothing else out
of this book, please retain this: You have a purpose in this life.
How do I know? You are here. That purpose was written on
your heart before you were born. Your job is to find that purpose and live it.

Before you throw this book across the room in frustration,
bear with me throughout the chapter. I know you may have
no idea what your life's purpose might be. Or maybe you have
an inkling of your purpose but are not sure how to live it. Or
perhaps you know your life's purpose but are stuck in a place
where you don't know if and how you can live it. Together

we will explore each of these scenarios and help you discover how to get closer to your dharma. But first, let me explain why dharma is so important.

The Importance of Dharma

Everything in existence has a dharma. Every single cell in your body has a dharma. A red blood cell would never try to become a brain cell, just as a tree would never try to become a flower. The manifestation of cancer cells occurs when normal cells "forget" their purpose.

It is my firm belief that most illness stems from our not living our life's purpose. When we are living out of sync with what we're supposed to be doing, our body feels it. We can, for a time, ignore our purpose, but sooner or later the body protests in an effort to get our attention. If we listen, chances are our body will heal. If we continue to ignore the signs, one of two things is likely to happen: either the illness we experience will become terminal, or modern medicine will assist us in healing for a time and we will experience a relapse later. Senior citizens who find a greater purpose in service after retirement offer an example of how a sense of purpose gives our bodies strength and greater health. Studies have shown that senior citizens with health problems who have a garden or a pet to care for become healthier.[1] This reality may sound harsh but it's true: If you have no higher purpose, you will die sooner than those who have one.

I had a client who was undergoing treatment for breast cancer. Two weeks after her retirement, she was diagnosed. For a year she went through surgery, chemotherapy, and radiation. I met her a few months into her treatment, and we then met weekly. After a couple of months with me, she told me about a huge project she was starting with her sister in order to serve humanity. With a glow in her eyes she said, "A lot of good has come out of my experience with cancer. My sister and I were not that close, and now we talk every day. I didn't know what I was going to do after retirement, and now I have this project." Chances are extremely good that she will permanently heal from her cancer. Among other changes she made in her life, she found a new life's purpose.

Dharma is inner drive, the tugging of the heartstrings that prompts you to live more fully. One person in the public eye who clearly demonstrates living in dharma is Diana Nyad. I recently heard her story on National Public Radio and was moved by her tenacity, passion, and drive. Nyad is the woman who, in 2013, at age sixty-four, swam from Havana, Cuba, to Key West, Florida, without a shark cage, in fifty-three hours. This was not Nyad's first attempt at making this particular swim, but her fifth attempt over the course of thirty-five years. She started her training for her most recent attempt at the 103-mile swim in 2010, and when a journalist asked her why, she responded, "Because I'd like to prove to other 60-year-olds that it is never too late to start your dreams."[2]

Your dharma will drive you to living it no matter what happens. Obstacles and delays may come your way. But if you are truly living your purpose, you will become unstoppable.

Defining Dharma

Have you ever come to a crossroads in your life where you have achieved many of your major goals, and where you recognize you are unhappy and that something must change? You obtained an education, found the love of your life, had a couple of kids, bought the car, the house, and the vacation home, and then, in a panic-stricken moment, looked around with discontent and said to yourself, "Now what?"

Over the course of our life, we often ask ourselves, "Why am I here?" "What am I supposed to be doing?" Or: "Now what?" Many times we ask this question in relation to a career, education choice, or goal. Most often, the question is linked to the financial outcome we expect to have when we have reached a goal or achievement. Unfortunately, most of us think of dharma, or purpose, in terms of something big, such as becoming a movie star or a sports hero. But it doesn't have to be quite so grandiose.

In the Indian tradition, the word *dharma*, although not easily translated, can be considered one's "righteous duty" or "virtuous path." For example, it is a bird's dharma to fly, a cow's dharma to produce milk, and a bee's dharma to make honey. It is your duty to live according to your dharma. And when you do, you are living in harmony with nature and the cosmos.

Being in harmony with the universe lets you feel like life is flowing. You have a sense of easily flowing downstream instead of constantly fighting your way up a current. All of us have experienced moments in our lives when we were "in the flow" or "living on purpose." Think back to the time when you first fell in love and this love was returned. For weeks and maybe months, you were floating on clouds, time had no bearing, and it didn't matter what the weather was like or who insulted you. You were in love. The whole world could come crashing down around you, and as long as you were with your beloved it didn't matter. Love is every person's dharma; and when you are in love, you have purpose. So does that mean we are to walk around with hearts and cupids all day? It might be interesting, but it might also get boring after a while. And we all know that the feeling of falling in love generally doesn't last forever. But that's the idea.

Other moments of flow you may have experienced might be scoring the winning basket for the final game in the season, baking the perfect cake, gazing into your baby's eyes for the first time, or leading a chorus in unison. These are what psychologist Abraham Maslow, in his *Religions, Values, and Peak-Experiences* (1964), referred to as "peak experiences." A peak experience is when time stands still, you are completely absorbed in the present moment, and whatever you are doing is effortless. You experience bliss and ease and recognize that the moment is right.

You may have many purposes in life; your purpose may change over time or develop in a way you never anticipated. Dharma does not have to be big in order to be meaningful. Living your dharma could entail raising children, being a bank teller, building houses, or picking up trash. If your work is effortless, you have a love for what you do, and you are in service of humanity, then you are in dharma. Other indications that you are in dharma are a sense of lightness in your body, a joyful or glowing feeling upon awakening in the morning, or a sense that time is flying by. I'm sure you've heard the expression "Time flies when you're having fun." When you are in dharma, your work is fun. Observe children at play, and you may notice that when a mother tries to take her child away from a highly creative playtime the child will protest. This is because the child is absorbed in the present moment. She is in dharma. Dr. Maria Montessori, the first Italian woman doctor and the originator of Montessori education, stated, "A child's play *is* his work." We can learn a lot from children about living in dharma.

We live in a world of overachievers. Western society teaches us that in order to be successful, we must get good grades, play an instrument, excel at a sport, be the president of a club or association, go to a top university, get the best salary at a Fortune 500 company, buy a big house, and drive an expensive car. And the list goes on. Do you get the picture? I live in northern Virginia, where competition is fierce, especially among children. There is a high school well known for its academic excellence in science and technology. It's a public school, but students must apply to get in. In 2011, over 3,000 students applied for 480 spots in the freshman class.

I heard a young girl explain that even with a perfect grade point average and awards in math and science, she still was not admitted. At fourteen years of age, this child was devastated because she did not get a spot in this competitive high school. She said that at her middle school she had been a math whiz and everyone knew it. Does the fact that she did not win admission to this school make her less intelligent in math? Will she fail to live her dharma if she does not attend this top school? I should think not. However, if she puts the fate of her love for math in someone else's hands and, for example, gives up studying math with a full heart, she will not be in dharma. Not everyone can fit the Western model of success I describe here; nor is it important. We are simply caught up in the belief that it's important. And the unfortunate consequence of this belief is that those who do not fit the model of Western success are often considered unsuccessful.

Recently a retired woman who was learning meditation with me explained that her husband of twenty-two years thought she was a failure because, according to him, she lived a "small life." To illustrate her point, she said, "I raised two boys, of whom I'm very proud, I was a manager at a large corporation, and I took care of my husband and the house. How could he say that I lived a 'small life'?" The sadness and frustration that emanated from her is a result of the disease that affects our society when it comes to the perception of success.

Finding Your Dharma

Imagine your life when you were a child about seven years old. Think of something you loved to do. Think of something you dreamed about doing. And think of something you said you were going to do when you grew up. This is a good age to reflect back on, because it precedes a lot of the social conditioning that would take place, but it's also an age that most of us can remember. Unfortunately, it may be a time, too, when the adults in your life gave you a little dose of "reality." If you expressed an interest in becoming a painter, Dad might have answered, "Well, that sounds nice, but how about getting a job that pays the bills?" Dharma would have been instantly crushed. Haven't we all heard phrases like: "Let's get practical," "Do something realistic," "Find a career that pays the bills," or "If I had pursued my interest in sports, would we be living in the house we have today?" So, as a seven-year-old who trusted your parents' advice, you put your dream aside and went on to study something more "practical." But maybe you still feel a tug inside to become a painter, dancer, or plumber. Now, I'm not suggesting you quit your job and become a full-time volunteer firefighter, if that's your dream. Unless you're independently wealthy, making the switch may not work for you and your family. What I *am* suggesting is that you begin the search for your dharma by asking yourself some questions.

Exercise: Discovering Dharma

Take a few minutes and complete the prompts in the following list. Be honest with yourself and don't hold back. Pretend you are a child again, or you're in another realm, one without limitations. If a desire or a theme continues to show up, be sure to write it down.

1. I love to:
2. My talents are:
3. Whenever I do the following, I lose track of time:
4. Things I could spend all day doing (eight hours or more) and not get bored or tired are:
5. If I could quit my job, I would:
6. My passions are:
7. I've always wanted to learn more about:
8. When I retire, I want to:
9. If money were no object, I would:
10. I like to serve others by doing:

Now read over your answers and circle any recurring themes. For example, if you answered, "I love to shop, and I lose track of time doing it," and "If I could quit my job, I would shop all day long," and "If money were no object, I would have a wardrobe full of fashionable clothing," then "shopping" is a recurring theme for you.

Once you've circled the recurring themes, take the top two, write them in the blanks provided, and fantasize a little. If you could invent the perfect job using these top two themes, what would it be? Write a paragraph for each one, describing in detail what the job would entail, what hours you would work each day, how many hours you would work, how much the job would pay, the location of your job (city, state, country, or actual company), and what your job description might look like. Don't stop or correct your spelling; write freely.

Theme 1:

Theme 2:

Now that you've finished the exercise, notice how you felt while creating your dream job. Notice the sensations in your body. Did you smile while writing it? Were you laughing? At some point, did you say to yourself, "I could actually do this"? Congratulate yourself for starting this exploration of dharma. You are on your way!

A Dose of Reality: When Doubt Creeps In

Social conditioning is not easy to overcome. And the reality is, we do have bills to pay, families to support, children to care for, and more. Perhaps you are naturally skeptical, so when that well-intentioned adult shut off your dreams when you were a child, you took it seriously and never dared to dream again. If in the exercise for inventing the perfect job you truly began to see your dharma, you may have felt a little sad inside because right now you can't see how to make it a reality. Or if you still have no idea what you're good at or where your passions or talents lie, you may be left frustrated or angry.

I Still Don't Know My Dharma

Honesty with yourself is a good place to begin the search for your dharma. If after doing the perfect-job exercise you cannot see your talents or passions, begin to observe yourself in different situations. Whenever you notice that a book, a TV show, or a conversation with someone has sparked your interest, observe your inner signals. Are you smiling, excited and intrigued to learn more? Does the topic make you think about something bigger than yourself? True dharma takes you beyond yourself into making others' lives better, brighter, happier, or more abundant. It does not mean you don't get pleasure from the work. But your own pleasure doesn't take precedence over all other considerations. Dharma often brings you to others rather than isolating you. It encourages you to realize that we are all connected. Remain aware that you're about to discover your life's purpose, and in time your hidden talents will surface.

I Know My Dharma but I Don't Know How to Make It a Reality

If you recognize your dharma but can't find a way to fulfill it, perhaps the direct translation of the word *dharma* from Sanskrit will help you. *Dharma* translates to "one's righteous duty or virtuous path." And not only do you have a calling, but you also have a duty to make living dharma a reality. No living creature on this planet, other than humans, questions its dharma. Can you imagine if a lion decided one day to become a vegetarian? And that this lion then encouraged other lions in its pride to stop hunting? A lion's dharma is to eat meat. By eating meat and being a hunter, it balances the ecosystem.

Let's suppose you've discovered that your true dharma is deep-sea scuba diving and teaching others how to scuba dive too. But you live in Ohio with your wife, three kids, and two dogs in a colonial-style house with a big mortgage. How, you might ask, can you even think of living your dharma without being irresponsible?

The answer is to find a new way to think about it. Maybe

you can save all your vacation days and put extra savings into a three- or four-week family vacation in a place where you can do deep-sea scuba diving each year. Or perhaps you can go to a place ideal for diving and invest in property there, which will allow you to live there after retirement. An even better solution might be to create your own company on the side, one that takes groups a couple of times a year on diving excursions, where you lead the group as an instructor and organizer and earn money in the process. The possibilities are absolutely endless. But you owe it to yourself and the rest of the world to live out your life's purpose while responsibly and faithfully fulfilling your other duties and obligations.

My Dharma Is Clear, but I Still Can't Take the Plunge

Knowing your dharma is exhilarating. It's exciting. But it doesn't mean you'll be fearless. Maybe for the first time ever, you're honoring your true nature. That's extremely scary because change is difficult, period. Acknowledge this and move on. In order to live according to your life's purpose you will, for some time, be living outside your comfort zone.

In 2006, I had been searching for my dharma for years. I had had inklings of my dharma. For example, I had known since I was small that writing was one of my life's purposes. And in 2001, right after September 11, I had taken on the blissful task of writing a book. After that, I wrote two novels and several children's books. I even spent a year writing to agents and publishing houses, but to no avail. So I continued to search. In a serendipitous event, I was led to teaching yoga, Ayurveda, and meditation. But let me emphasize that it was not easy, ever. In the two years after I made the decision, in 2006, to pursue this path, I got divorced and moved from France back to Virginia with my three kids, two cats, and no job or career. I had decided to start my Ayurvedic business without any business experience whatsoever. Everyone around me thought I was crazy. When money didn't come in on time or when the business got rough in some other way, I even began to doubt myself. But deep down I knew this was my path. I just knew it.

Please don't get me wrong: knowing doesn't mean you won't have periods of self-doubt and uncertainty. When that happens, go to your heart space. Take a day and look inside yourself for the truth. No one but you knows your truth. Live that truth and place your trust in it. If the way you're pursuing your dharma is not working, then change direction. But I cannot emphasize enough that you must take the plunge. You do not want to reach the end of your life and say to yourself, "I wish I would have…" or "I should have…"

Intention and Desire: Creating Your Life's Purpose

One way to get clear on dharma is to create a list of your intentions and desires. This is a bit different from setting goals, because it has a component of surrender. Often when we have a goals list and we don't complete it, or the goals don't turn out as planned, we are disappointed, frustrated, or angry. In creating intention, we acknowledge our desires with words, visualization, and intent, but we are trusting that the outcome will unfold according to universal plan. I understand this is not an easy thing to do. Admitting that you don't have total control over the outcome isn't something we've been taught to do, especially in the United States. One of the interesting things about growing up in a monotheistic faith such as Christianity, Judaism, or Islam is that followers are taught the principle of surrender, as in the expression "Let go and let God." However, cultural conditioning, in the United States at least, overrides this concept as we become goal oriented and driven while living the American dream. Even if you don't believe in God or a higher being, if you sit and observe nature for a time you will notice a perfect orchestration of universal energy. There's something bigger at play here. Watch a flock of birds soaring through the sky, turning in formation with exact precision. Human pilots trying to do the same thing have to work at it for years, but birds do it effortlessly.

Observe trees as they turn from seemingly dead pieces of wood in winter to living, blossoming specimens in the spring. We too are a part of nature, the perfect orchestration of the universe. Somehow, through our thought processes, we lose our way and our connection to the conductor. In chapter 4, we will discuss ways of reconnecting to the impulse within you, an impulse that is also in the butterflies, the trees, and the plants.

For the sake of expanding your understanding of dharma now, it is important to take this step of setting your intentions and listing your desires. What is it that you desire? Desires are not wrong; they aren't to be snuffed out with shame or self-doubt. Some desires serve a higher purpose than others, but as your awareness evolves and grows, so too will your desires.

A desire can be anything that takes into account the values of gratitude, honesty, integrity, love, forgiveness, and trust. The universe wants balance and harmony, so any desire that is disharmonious with the overall well-being of the universe is unlikely to be manifested. So if on your list you write, "I want my mother-in-law to be hit by a car," you are not obeying the universal law of love. And even if your wish were to come true, you would only bring negative karmic energy into your life — and that's not what you wish to accomplish.

A desire doesn't have to be selfless as long as it includes the values listed in the preceding paragraph. For example, let's say you desire a BMW convertible. If you acquire the car honestly and with integrity (for example, by not stealing the money for it), and you keep love and gratitude in your heart in the process, your desire will bring positive energy to your life and maintain the harmony of the universe. But if you take that car and use it to sell drugs or drive recklessly on the highway, putting others' lives in danger, you will create an imbalance in the universe as you fulfill your desire.

Writing down an intention presupposes that the object of your desire is already here, because it is. You just haven't found a way to see it yet. Suppose your dream job is one that will pay a hundred thousand dollars a year, give you four weeks' vacation annually, allow you to work from home two days a week, and require only a five-mile commute or less. A job like that certainly exists. You need to set your intention and know that it will manifest in your life at the appropriate time.

Be specific about your desire. The idea here is to be specific but not rigid. If you are too vague, you will not recognize the direction you must take. If you're too rigid, you will eliminate better possibilities that you aren't able to see now. Instead of saying, "I want a new house," give some specifics. For example: "It is my intention to manifest a new house with four bedrooms, two and a half baths, a sunny kitchen, and a finished basement, located on a calm street with a cul-de-sac."

Take action in the direction you want to go. Once you write down your intention, don't just sit back and wait for manna to fall from heaven. To use the example of the house: do some research, contact real estate agents, get your finances in order, get preapproved for a mortgage, and visit houses that correspond to your intention. During the process, you are trusting that the universe really will handle the details.

Be open to the unexpected; avoid putting on blinders. Usually when we set a goal, we have in mind a certain picture of how we'd like it to turn out. We even anticipate the path that it will take. Visualization is a fantastic tool in the process of manifesting intentions, but stay on the lookout for unexpected opportunities. If we remain set in our ways, we may not see a different open road that appears before us. Consider every phone call, email, meeting, or conversation a possibility for getting what you desire, even when things don't go your way. The truth is, you never know exactly how the process of reaching your goal will unfold. For example, if your car breaks down on the highway, and you have to wait all day at the car dealership for it to be fixed, you may have the opportunity to meet a person in the waiting room who can fulfill your desire.

I have a habit of keeping a list of my intentions and a list of my manifested intentions. When an intention manifests, I switch it to the other list and add a brief explanation of how it manifested. This is a reminder to myself that I don't always understand how it works, but that it does. Develop a sense of gratitude for what you do have. It helps attract into your life what you desire. Always say thank you in the morning for everything in your life.

Exercise: List of Intentions and Desires

Start by making a list of your ten greatest intentions and desires. Your intentions can relate to any aspect of your life. As you see your intentions come to fruition, create a "manifested intentions" list, which explains how and when each intention came to be in your life.

✔ Checklist for Health

Dharma

❑ Complete the exercise on exploring your dharma.

❑ Find the recurring themes in your life that surround your passions.

❑ Throughout your week, look for clues to what gives you bliss or creates that inner spark.

❑ Create your list of intentions and desires. Make copies, and keep a copy with you. Put a copy in a place where you will see it every day, and put a copy in a place where you meditate. Read your list daily.

❑ Make a commitment to yourself to explore, do, or plan one thing that will get you closer to living your dharma.

❑ Start a "manifested intentions" list, and begin to watch the magic unfold as your intentions become reality.

CHAPTER THREE

PHYSICAL HEALTH

Let food be thy medicine and medicine be thy food.

— HIPPOCRATES

Often when we think of our health, we mainly focus on the physical body. Starting with the body is a good beginning point, since so much of what we do daily either adds to or subtracts from our physical health. Ayurveda gives us many tools to balance our bodies, including diet, daily routine, and an exercise program.

Food as Medicine

The adage "You are what you eat" is more than a cliché. More than ever, in today's world, it's a reality. And what we have available to eat is increasingly artificial, genetically modified, chemical laden, and simply unhealthy. Even though the choices may seem varied, in actuality they're limited to a few ingredients, which show up in different products. So what should you eat to maintain optimal health?

First, I'd like you to consider a few facts and natural inclinations we have. This will put you in touch with your intuitive nature. Fact no. 1: We need to eat in order to stay alive. Fact no. 2: Our ancestors, who lived before the Industrial Revolution, had to rely on hunting, gathering, growing, and storing food to survive. Fact no. 3: Because the human body has been hardwired over time for survival, eating large amounts of food or yo-yo dieting will lead to weight gain.

In the postindustrial era, processed or chemically produced food has become the norm. Owing to shrewd and manipulative advertising, most people don't even know the difference between something healthy and something processed. If one cereal carries the claim that it will lower cholesterol and is endorsed by the American Heart Association, why shouldn't we believe it? If a yogurt company makes the claim that their yogurt has five grams of fiber, and your doctor says you must get more fiber, why not buy that yogurt? One thing we need to realize is that advertisers tell partial truths. Food manufacturers and distributors are multibillion-dollar corporations. If you don't believe their claims, their advertising teams are doing a poor job. In 2010, Kraft Food's net revenue was $49.2 billion. In comparison, smaller, organic food companies, such as Horizon Organic Dairy, bring in around $50 to $100 million in net revenue. It's not surprising that we believe the large food companies' claims, given how loud and how present they are in our daily lives.

For millions of years, humans have eaten what was available from the earth; and for the past one hundred years or so, they've eaten what's available. Do you understand the difference in that statement? In order to obtain optimal health, we need to go back to eating what's available from the earth, because that is what we're hardwired to process. Biological evolution takes a great number of generations, not one or two generations. By pouring chemically produced food and drink into our bodies, we are attempting to force biological evolution over the period of one lifetime. And our bodies are protesting. According to the World Health Organization, world cancer rates could increase by 50 percent, to 15 million new cases by 2020.[1] And according to the Centers for Disease Control, obesity is the number two preventable cause of death in the United States.[2]

Poor diet costs us not only our lives but our resources as well. Type 2 diabetes, a completely preventable form of diabetes, drains $63.14 billion from our health care system yearly, and that figure doesn't take into account the cost of lost days of work, physician office visits, and the detriment to families. Close runners-up in preventable disease are hypertension and heart disease, followed by osteoarthritis and gallbladder disease.

The good news is that you can do something about all this. With a shift in awareness and a change in habits, you get to take control of your health and life. Most people only dabble in a healthy lifestyle and then brace themselves for a cancer diagnosis or for some other disease that may creep up. But most diseases don't "come out of nowhere." Disease is developed over years and sometimes decades. According to Ayurvedic medicine, 95 percent of diseases are completely preventable with a consistent, proper lifestyle, one that includes a good diet, meditation, and an exercise regime. This is good news because you are in control. Being in control means you take responsibility for your own health. Leaving your health to doctors, medicines, other health care practitioners, or fate means leaving the door wide open to greater health problems in the future. When it comes to health, there is a place for allopathic medicine, herbal medicine, and, yes, prayer, but those are certainly not ways to prevent ill health. They are simply bandages applied to what's already broken.

What I'm emphasizing here is taking real responsibility on a daily basis, starting now, today. There's a reason why you picked up this book, and this is it. By taking responsibility, you cannot blame anyone or anything for your sickness or disease. I understand that you may be reluctant to take full responsibility, because doing so requires effort and additional resources. Here are some of the excuses that I hear in my practice:

- I don't have the time.
- I don't have the money.
- I don't have the motivation.
- My husband, wife, significant other, roommate, mother, or father keeps unhealthy food in the house, so I can't eat healthfully.
- I live in a rural area, so there are no health stores nearby.
- I'm lazy.
- I have to take care of everyone else; I can't take time for myself.
- I'm too tired at the end of the day.

Let me address these excuses one by one and prove to you that taking responsibility is necessary regardless of any excuses you may have.

I Don't Have the Time

Everyone has twenty-four hours in a day. How is it that some people are able to accomplish much, while others are chasing the clock? What takes time? Going to the grocery store? Cooking? Working out? Let me ask you this: How much time do you spend watching TV? Surfing the Internet? Texting? Doing tasks that others can do for you? Can you spend fewer hours doing these things and more hours taking care of your health?

There are ways to integrate your family and others into your healthy lifestyle. Get your kids to plan meals, cook, and clean up with you. Have a date night with your significant other, where you cook a healthy meal together. Watch your favorite TV show while working out on the treadmill. Call your best friend while you're out jogging. Integrate tasks with exercise and cooking, and you will save time.

I Don't Have the Money

Do you have the money to take time off from work when you need to stay home because you're sick, or when you need chemo treatments or surgery? Do you have the money to fork out for copayments for doctor visits, prescription drugs, and the lost family time that you can never get back? Besides, not having money is a myth, because we all have to eat. With planning, you may even save money because you won't be snacking on a bunch of empty calories and your body will be filled with the good stuff. Since you'll eat only what you need, and you won't cook in excess, you'll buy less food each week. But let's face it, a healthy lifestyle is an investment. It is an investment more valuable than your house, your car, your wardrobe, your electronic devices, and your retirement fund.

Without your health, what do you have? Seriously, answer that question: What will you have without your health? The answer is: nothing. For a time, you may have your family or friends, but they will move on with their lives. And if they see that you are not taking care of yourself, they will begin to resent you for taking advantage of their kindness. If you don't have your health, can you maintain a job, hobbies, and social activities? If you don't have your health, how can you volunteer and serve your community? If you're too sick to enjoy anything, it won't matter whether you have your own house, a car, electronics, or fancy clothes. Does that sound painful? Well, it should. Because it is. You can't afford to not invest in your health.

I Don't Have the Motivation

Hopefully, after reading the discussion of excuse no. 2 you're motivated. But if you're not, think of all the reasons you're here on earth and list them now. And if those reasons aren't motivating enough, list others. The shift you're beginning to make is toward the belief that your body is the temple that houses your soul. Everything in life that is near and dear to you is experienced only with your body, through your senses. Without your body, you can't experience life on earth.

The body, therefore, is sacred. It's not just a place to dump a bunch of calories regardless of their origin. It is a miracle to be celebrated daily. If you knew the miracle of the body, you would be in awe every single day. With 60 trillion to 90 trillion cells acting in concert all the time to keep you healthy, it's a wonder that we're not sick more often. After treating the body unkindly, with Pop-Tarts, Pringles, or three-day-old pizza and a soda, we berate the body for getting the flu or a cold. Imagine your body retorting with: "Hey, I'm trying my best here with the resources you're giving me."

My Husband, Wife, Significant Other, Roommate, Mother, or Father Keeps Unhealthy Food in the House, So I Can't Eat Healthfully

This excuse brings up the question of taking responsibility for *your* health. You aren't responsible for the health of others, with the exception of your children; and even then, they are ultimately responsible for their health since you can't be with them twenty-four hours a day. Sometimes you don't have control over the food in the house, in the workplace, or at social gatherings. You do, however, have control over what you put into your mouth every single time. If someone else is doing the cooking, ask to take over that task or teach him or her how to cook using the new guidelines you will learn in this chapter. Remember, you are in control. This is your body, your life. However, please be kind to the people in your life as you're making this shift. Think about how long it took you to come to this point. The best way to get others on board is not only to be enthusiastic about what you're learning but also to let them see the results of these healthy practices in your body, mind, and energy level.

I Live in a Rural Area, So There Are No Health Stores Nearby

I understand this problem completely. When traveling, I sometimes encounter difficulty in finding organic produce and other healthy products. It's frustrating. With the increased interest in healthy eating, the demand for healthier products in rural areas will rise — and it already has. This is the basic principle of supply and demand. The more consumers demand organic, non–genetically modified products, the more producers will provide them. But simultaneously, consumers must stop buying junk food, so companies will see a decline in their revenues and ask themselves what's wrong. Money talks, and that's the only way consumers can gain the power to decide what's on the shelves.

If you live in a rural area, you have some advantages. The air you're breathing may be better than in the city or suburbs. You may have more space for walks and jogs. You likely have access to farmers' markets and roadside fresh-produce stands. And you may have the space to start your own organic garden. So look at the upside. If it's other products you're worried about, such as organic grains, cereals, nuts, and meats, you may have to do your homework. Costco Wholesale sells many organic products, including olive oil, brown rice, and milk. Even if the nearest Costco is an hour or two away, you can stock up on dry staples that will last you for some time. Online stores may be another source. If you plan meals and know what you use the most, you may find it necessary to order and pay shipping costs only once or twice a month. But it is my hope that the shift now taking place will happen on a global level as we begin to change the marketplace.

I'm Lazy

It's no wonder you're lazy. If you've been filling your body with everything except what it needs, how can you expect it to work properly? Would you fill your car with cooking oil to save time and money? Laziness is a by-product of a sedentary lifestyle, a symptom you're experiencing, and not your nature. Follow an Ayurvedic lifestyle, including the diet outlined for you here, for twenty-one days straight and see if laziness is a problem. I challenge you!

I Have to Take Care of Everyone Else; I Can't Take Time for Myself

Change that thought to: "I must take care of myself before I can take care of anyone else." Copy this statement and tape it to your bathroom mirror, your bedpost, your car's dashboard, your computer screen — everywhere. If you've ever been on an airplane, you know that the flight attendant instructs you to put on your *own* mask before assisting others in the case of cabin-pressure loss. Need I say more? Unfortunately, mothers most often make this excuse. I can relate to this completely because I was there too. I felt guilty at times (and still do) when I took time away from my kids or significant other to exercise, cook healthy meals, or meditate. But let me tell you this, if you're a mother: you cannot give your children a better or more beautiful gift than to portray to them, through your actions, that health is the number one priority. Children may not listen to what you say, but they follow what you do.

I'm Too Tired at the End of the Day

If that's the case, start your day with exercise, chop vegetables in the morning, and make that vegetarian chili or soup in a slow cooker. You don't have to do it all at the end of the day. With planning you can also sneak exercise in during the workday.

I always ask my Ayurvedic clients whether their jobs give them a lunch break. The answer is always yes. My next question is: Do you take your lunch break? The answer most often is no. And then I follow it with: "If you took your lunch break, would you get fired?" The answer is no. Then I say, "Well, could you take your one-hour lunch break and walk for one hour, or jog, or go to the gym, and then eat lunch at your desk like you normally do?" The answer is either yes or "yes, but." The "yes, but" is: "Yes, but I'll get sweaty." "Yes, but people might look at me weird if I take a break," or something similar. My reply to that is: Be a leader in this movement. Recruit your fellow employees to walk with you. It doesn't matter if there's no trail; walk the parking lot. Form a lunchtime walking club, recruit your boss, suggest a walk-and-talk meeting outdoors. Take a sponge bath in the bathroom afterward. Who cares if you're a little sweaty? Bring some deodorant to work. In other words, the possibilities are endless. If there's a will, there most certainly is a way.

An Ayurvedic Plan for Optimal Nutrition

There are a few steadfast rules about nutrition in an Ayurvedic lifestyle. Most of these represent a commonsense approach to healthy eating as a whole. When I teach my Ayurvedic lifestyle course, I emphasize the 90–10 rule, which means you may implement the nutritional guidelines 90 percent of the time and allow yourself 10 percent flexibility in your daily diet. In the beginning these guidelines may seem rigid or extreme, but they are less extreme than many of the weight-loss schemes in mainstream society, and they don't exclude any major food groups. Once you integrate these guidelines into your daily life, it will be difficult to go back to the way you ate previously, because your body will begin to feel fantastic and you won't want to lose that feeling. But the rules are meant to guide you back to health, not make you crazy. There's a wise saying in Indian philosophy that states, "Infinite flexibility is the key to immortality." So, when applying the guidelines, keep in mind that deviating from time to time is okay and may even be healthy, because with flexibility you can enjoy life more. So go ahead and eat your grandmother's mincemeat pie, or drink that milkshake from your favorite ice cream shop. But do it with awareness and enjoyment, and don't overdo it. Remember the 90–10 rule.

The Twelve Guidelines
for an Ayurvedic Lifestyle Eating Plan

1. Eat freshly prepared foods at every meal.
2. Choose organic and locally grown produce and grains whenever available.
3. Choose only organic grass-fed dairy, eggs, poultry, and meat.
4. Eat all six tastes at every meal: sweet, sour, salty, bitter, pungent, and astringent.
5. Reduce your consumption of packaged and processed foods.

6. Choose the five *sattvic*, or healing, foods in their organic form whenever possible: milk, ghee, almonds, honey, fruit.

7. Let vegetables and fruit make up 50 to 60 percent of your daily food intake.

8. Eliminate unhealthy oils: hydrogenated or partially hydrogenated oils, margarine, and shortening.

9. Eliminate high-fructose corn syrup; other types of corn syrup; artificial sweeteners; bleached, enriched flour; and white, processed sugar.

10. Reduce your consumption of frozen and canned food.

11. Drink filtered, distilled, or spring water.

12. Be moderate and avoid extremes.

1. Eat Freshly Prepared Foods at Every Meal

I understand that this rule may turn you upside down. American cooking has emphasized using leftovers or making meals ahead of time and freezing them. If you're from a different culture, the concept of eating only freshly prepared foods may not seem so foreign to you.

When we think about nourishing our bodies, we must think about optimal nutrition on all levels. We're only as healthy as the cells that make up our body, and so we need to offer our body food that contains the most nutrients in every bite. Let me clarify that we are not talking about calories here. As Americans, we are overly focused on the number of calories when we should be focused on the quality of the calories. In order to create healthy cells, our bodies must be able to extract the nutrients — phytonutrients, vitamins, minerals, amino acids, and so on — from the food we ingest. The fresher the foods, the more of these nutrients they contain. After a food is cooked or picked, or even worse, once it's been processed, the food begins to decompose and loses its nutritional value. Here's my rule of thumb: eat the prepared food within twenty-four hours of making it. This requires you to cook less food and prepare it more often; but with the exception of certain curry dishes and marinated salads, fresh food tastes better anyway.

2. Choose Organic and Locally Grown Produce and Grains Whenever Available

Organic fruit, vegetables, grains, and even meat can be found in most grocery stores and supermarkets today. An important component of Ayurvedic nutrition is to minimize the amount of toxins entering the body and maximize the number of nutrients. Organically grown food is grown without synthetic pesticides (including herbicides) and synthetic fertilizers and is free of genetic modifications. As a consequence, organic foods are higher in antioxidants and phytonutrients and lower in toxins. Furthermore, by keeping harmful chemicals out of our soil and water supply, organic food helps to keep our earth healthy. And in general, organic food tastes better.

When it's not possible to buy organic produce, the next best option is conventionally grown local produce. Check out a nearby farmers' market and talk to the farmers. Ask them what their practices are regarding pesticides and synthetic fertilizers. Many farmers will say they operate a "no spray" farm but cannot receive the USDA organic label because it's too costly for a smaller farm. This doesn't necessarily mean these local farmers are growing organic produce, but it may be a good option when organic produce is not available. Another option for buying produce is to join a food co-op. During the spring and summer, many farms offer co-op programs where you can purchase a box of produce weekly. Depending on the program, you may be able to choose what's in the box, and you're

guaranteed fresh produce each week. Go to www.localharvest
.org/organic-farms/ to find a co-op program near you.

3. Choose Only Organic Grass-Fed Dairy, Eggs, Poultry, and Meat

In addition to being fed plants treated with pesticides and grown
from genetically modified seeds, feedlot animals are given anti-
biotics and growth hormones to maximize and speed up their
growth and keep them alive. Dairy cows are given a genetically
engineered hormone, rBGH, to increase milk production. And
most cows, who are meant to eat grass and clover, are fed a
grain-based diet. Unless you have your own cow, the best way to
ensure that you're getting the best dairy products possible is to
choose grass-fed dairy products. One of the best dairy-product
lines I've found is Natural by Nature. Find distributors of this
company's products at www.natural-by-nature.com. If you eat
beef, you can also find grass-fed beef in organic markets.

When choosing organic eggs, make sure they are USDA
certified organic. And go with the better-known brands, such
as Vital Farms, Organic Valley, and Horizon Organic. Be wary
of phrases on labels such as "natural," "farm raised," and "free
range." While these words may be enticing, they do not hold
the farmer accountable with respect to organic and sustainable
practices.

4. Eat All Six Tastes at Every Meal: Sweet, Sour, Salty, Bitter, Pungent, and Astringent

In Ayurveda, foods are composed of six tastes: sweet, sour, salty,
bitter, pungent, and astringent. Any given food has a primary, or
baseline, taste and may also have a secondary and even a tertiary
taste. A good example of this is meat: the baseline taste of meat is

sweet, but its secondary taste is salty. According to Ayurveda, we must receive all six tastes at every meal for optimal nutrition and to minimize cravings and prevent overeating. Once you learn how to integrate the six tastes in every meal, you will see the spikes and valleys in your hunger level out.

In the audio program *Magical Mind, Magical Body*, Dr. Deepak Chopra points out that animals in the forest don't have the faintest idea of what the USDA has to say about the food pyramid or of its recommendations for vitamin and mineral intake, yet they don't have nutritional deficiencies. The only species that becomes nutritionally deficient is the human species. And we do so because we've completely lost touch with the inner wisdom of our bodies. As we start to heal and attune ourselves to our bodies' needs, we begin to know exactly what they need. Have you ever finished a meal and felt dissatisfied? It may have felt that something was missing but you couldn't put your finger on it. By getting all six tastes at every meal, you will be continually fulfilling your body's need for specific nutrients, and so you will be less likely to over-eat or eat the wrong kinds of food. This concept is unique to Ayurveda and truly helps diminish and eventually eliminate cravings.

SWEET: The first taste is sweet and is found in protein, fat, and carbohydrates. In the West when we think of the sweet taste, we generally associate it with sugary products like candy and ice cream. In Ayurveda, meat, oils, and butter are sweet. Milk, too, is sweet, as are cereals, other grains, and sweet fruit.

SOUR: The second taste is sour and is the taste of citrus fruits and fermented foods and drinks, such as yogurt, sour cream, cheese, vinegar, and alcohol.

SALTY: The third taste on our list, salty, presumably doesn't require further explanation; it is easy to receive in food.

BITTER: The fourth taste is bitter and is most often found in leafy greens or vegetables.

PUNGENT: The fifth taste, pungent, is the taste of spice or peppery heat. Pungency is found in such foods as spices, hot peppers, garlic, onions, and ginger.

ASTRINGENT: The sixth taste, astringent, is not a true taste but nonetheless must be included. Foods that possess astringent taste have a peculiar flavor and have a compacting and drying effect on the body. Some examples are beans, lentils, and pulses but also green tea, spinach, and cranberries. If you've ever had a cup of pure green tea without anything added to it, you have experienced a dry taste in your mouth. That is the effect of astringency.

Since only a small quantity of foods with bitter, pungent, or astringent tastes is necessary to satisfy our requirements, it's relatively easy to include them in your daily diet. For example, a couple of dashes of pepper will add the pungency, while a small amount of raw spinach in a salad will give you the bitter and astringent tastes.

Below is a list of common foods in each taste category. This list is a guide and, while it doesn't include every food, it can help you determine which foods you can eat more of to help you balance your dosha. Keep in mind that most foods have a dominant taste but also a secondary taste. Some foods have more than two tastes. For example, apples' primary taste is sweet, and their secondary taste is astringent. When filling your plate, try to include foods from each of the six taste categories.

The Six Tastes — Common Foods

SWEET

Almonds
Apples (except green)
Apricots
Artichokes*
Asparagus*
Avocados*
Bananas
Barley
Beets
Black beans*
Brazil nuts
Bread
Buckwheat*
Butter
Cardamom
Carrots
Cashews
Celery*
Cherries
Cilantro*
Cinnamon
Coconut
Corn
Cucumbers
Dates
Dill
Eggs
Fava beans
Fennel
Figs
Filberts
Fish, freshwater
Ghee
Grains
Grapes, purple
Green beans*
Guava
Honey
Ice cream
Lentils*
Lima beans*

Macadamias
Mangoes
Meats
Melons
Milk
Millet
Mint
Mung beans*
Mushrooms*
Navy beans*
Nutmeg
Oats
Oils, all
Okra
Onions, cooked
Oranges
Papayas
Pasta
Peaches
Peanuts
Pears
Peas*
Pecans
Peppers, bell
Persimmons
Pine nuts
Pineapples
Pistachios
Plums
Pomegranates
Poppy seeds
Potatoes*
Pumpkin seeds
Rice
Sesame seeds
Spices, sweet
Squash
Strawberries*
Sugar
Sunflower seeds
Sweet potatoes
Tangerines

Tomatoes, yellow
Walnuts
Wheat
Yogurt

SOUR

Alcohol
Apples, green
Apricots*
Berries
Caraway
Cheese
Cherries*
Cottage cheese
Cranberries
Grapefruit
Grapes, green
Kefir cheese
Lemons
Limes
Oranges*
Oregano
Papaya*
Pickles
Pineapples*
Plums*
Sour cream
Strawberries
Tomatoes, red
Vinegar
Yogurt*

SALTY

Braggs Liquid Aminos
Celery*
Fish, ocean*
Meats*
Salt
Sea veggies
Soy sauce
Tamari

The Six Tastes — Common Foods

PUNGENT

Alcohol*
Asafetida
Basil
Bay leaves
Caraway
Cayenne
Chamomile
Cloves
Coffee
Eggplant
Fennel
Fenugreek
Garbanzo beans
Garlic
Ginger
Marjoram
Mustard, grain
Mustard greens*
Mustard oil
Nutmeg*
Onions, raw
Parsley*
Pepper, black
Peppers, chili
Pumpkin seeds*
Radishes
Rosemary
Thyme
Turmeric
Turnips

BITTER

Almonds*
Aloe vera
Asparagus
Bitter melons
Broccoli*
Chamomile
Chard
Coffee

Eggplant*
Greens, leafy
Kale
Limes*
Mustard, grain*
Mustard greens
Rosemary
Spinach
Tea
Turmeric*
Veggies, yellow

ASTRINGENT

Alfalfa sprouts
Apples* (all)
Artichokes
Asparagus
Avocados
Bananas*
Barley*
Berries*
Bean (mung) sprouts
Broccoli
Brussels sprouts
Buckwheat
Cabbage
Carrots*
Cauliflower
Celery
Cilantro
Corn
Cranberries
Cucumbers*
Dill
Eggplant*
Figs*
Fish, fresh
Green beans
Greens, dark leafy*
Jerusalem artichokes
Kidney beans

Lemons*
Lentils
Lettuce
Lima beans
Mushrooms
Nutmeg*
Okra
Oregano
Parsley
Peaches*
Pears*
Peas
Peppers, bell*
Plums*
Pomegranates*
Potatoes*
Radishes*
Rice*
Sea veggies*
Sesame seeds*
Soy/tofu (natural forms in unprocessed foods)
Spinach*
Split peas
Squash*
Strawberries
Tea, green
Turmeric*
Turnips*
Wheat*

* Secondary tastes

SAMPLE MEALS THAT INCLUDE ALL SIX TASTES

VATA-PACIFYING BREAKFAST: Cream of wheat with milk (sweet) made with a pinch of salt (salty), sweetened with maple syrup (sweet), and topped with berries or cherries (sour) and a dash of cinnamon and nutmeg (pungent). Accompany this with a cup of green tea (bitter and astringent).

PITTA-PACIFYING LUNCH: A spinach salad (bitter and astringent) with sliced avocados (astringent and sweet), sunflower seeds (sweet), olive oil (sweet), vinegar (sour), salt and pepper (salty and pungent), sprouts (astringent), and cucumbers (sweet and astringent).

KAPHA-PACIFYING DINNER: Stir-fried tofu (astringent and sweet) with broccoli (bitter and astringent), garlic (pungent), celery (salty and astringent), pineapple (sour and sweet), kale (bitter), sesame oil (sweet and astringent), brown rice (sweet), and soy sauce (salty).

5. Reduce Your Consumption of Packaged and Processed Foods

If you must use processed foods, observe the following:

- Choose packaged products labeled "USDA Organic."
- Choose products with no more than six ingredients listed on the label; and you must know what the ingredients are and what food source they come from.

6. Choose the Five Sattvic, or Healing, Foods in Their Organic Form Whenever Possible: Milk, Ghee, Almonds, Honey, Fruit

There are a few exceptions to this rule. Kapha types and those who are on Kapha-pacifying diets must minimize their consumption of milk, ghee, and honey. Diabetics need to closely monitor their consumption of honey and fruit owing to the high sugar content. Milk is revered in Ayurveda as a complete food. It should be brought to the boiling point first and then cooled slightly before drinking. Warmed milk combined with a teaspoon of ghee has a mild laxative effect and can be used to treat constipation or sluggish bowels. Warm milk with cardamom, nutmeg, and a teaspoon of sugar can induce sleep when taken in the evening. If you are calcium deficient or are at risk for osteoporosis, soak ten almonds overnight and peel and eat them in the morning.

7. Let Vegetables and Fruit Make Up 50 to 60 Percent of Your Daily Food Intake

Ayurvedic medicine presupposes a vegetarian diet. However, if this is not desirable or possible, strive to make vegetables and fruits at least 50 percent of your daily food intake. This is necessary because these are water-rich foods, and our bodies are 50 to 65 percent water and our brains are 85 percent water. By eating water-rich foods, you are sure to get enough water in your body; most people don't consume enough water to stay hydrated. The second reason is that phytonutrients, which protect us from cancer, heart disease, and premature aging, are found only in plants. Third, antioxidants, or free-radical scavengers, which help repair damaged cells and prevent cancer growth, are found mostly in plant-based foods.

8. Eliminate Unhealthy Oils: Hydrogenated or Partially Hydrogenated Oils, Margarine, and Shortening

Favor organic olive oil, canola oil, sesame oil, and butter in your diet, because they are higher-quality oils and fats. During the fat-free craze that began in the 1980s, butter was given a bad rap. Organic butter is a saturated fat but is okay to eat

in moderation and certainly better to eat than chemically prepared butter substitutes.

9. Eliminate High-Fructose Corn Syrup; Other Types of Corn Syrup; Artificial Sweeteners; Bleached, Enriched Flour; and White, Processed Sugar

Because of our genetic blueprints passed down from our
ancestors, our bodies are hardwired to recognize natural foods
and know what to do with them. High-fructose corn syrup
was developed in 1967, and our bodies have hardly had time to
adjust to this product and learn what to do with it. Chemically
engineered artificial sweeteners are known to cause a spike
in insulin levels, which may tire out the pancreas. Bleached,
enriched flour is actually stripped of its nutritional value: the
germ and outer bran layers are removed and the wheat is then
bleached with oxide of nitrogen, chlorine, chloride, nitrosyl,
and benzoyl peroxide mixed with various chemical salts. Using
this flour means that you not only consume something devoid
of nutrients but also ingest residual chemicals. Instead of eating any of these products, choose organic, unbleached, un-
bromated flour and organic turbinado sugar, organic sugar,
organic brown sugar, organic honey, and organic grade A
maple syrup.

10. Reduce Your Consumption of Frozen and Canned Food

When the variety of fresh produce is limited at certain times
of the year, is frozen produce better? When it comes to nutrients, time is of the essence. The longer a plant-based food has
been out of the ground, or the longer an animal-based food
has been dead, the fewer nutrients it contains. There is a principle in Ayurveda called *prana*, or "life force and vitality." A

living thing has prana unless it has been altered by chemicals, laden with toxins, or deprived of sunlight and water. The same prana in a living entity is given to us in food. As soon as a plant is pulled from the earth or an animal is slaughtered for meat, it begins to lose its prana and continues to lose it as the days go by. Food that has been frozen is literally prana frozen in time, but eventually that food loses its prana. How much prana is present in frozen food depends on the length of time it has been frozen. Most canned food has been preserved in water or some other liquid, and the nutrients leak into the liquid while the can sits on the shelf. And since most of us throw away the liquid surrounding the food, we toss out the nutrients as well. As a rule of thumb, if your food hasn't seen sunlight in a while, it's best to reduce your consumption of that food or eliminate it from your diet altogether.

11. Drink Filtered, Distilled, or Spring Water

Water is, without a doubt, the most important thing we put into our bodies. Given that our bodies are about two-thirds water and our brains are over 80 percent water, it's no wonder we feel cranky when we're even slightly dehydrated. The minimum amount of water you should drink daily is eight eight-ounce glasses. It's best not to count beverages such as tea, coffee, or soda as part of that amount. They have a diuretic effect on the body, causing you to urinate more frequently and, in doing so, lose water more rapidly than normal. People with a larger body mass, and athletic people, may need additional water.

Ideally, drink half your body weight in ounces. For example, if you weigh 140 pounds, then strive to drink 70 ounces of water. If taste is an issue, add a few drops of fresh lemon or lime juice or a few tablespoons of other natural juice to the water.

Many clients tell me they forget to drink water. My advice is to fill a container with the amount of water you need to drink for the day and take it from there.

Water quality is extremely important. Most tap water is heavily chlorinated or has other chemicals meant to keep it free of microorganisms. Distilled water is likely to be the safest. Spring water would be a good choice too. Filtered water may improve taste, but not all filters remove contaminants.

12. Be Moderate and Avoid Extremes

Remember the 90–10 rule: implement the nutritional guidelines 90 percent of the time and allow yourself 10 percent flexibility. My dear teacher Dr. David Simon often said, "If you say 'do not' or 'cannot' too many times, it will tie you in knots." Follow the guidelines most of the time, and they will become a part of who you are. But don't go crazy. Eat ice cream once in a while; have a frozen pizza. Just don't let that become the norm.

Guidelines for Re-creating the Mind-Body Connection with Food

Awareness comes on all levels. Food awareness is important in reconnecting the body-mind. If you've ever tried to feed a young child, you know that it's a struggle to get him to eat when he's not hungry. Certain food, situations, emotions, environments, or circumstances can create a disconnect between the body and the mind and soul when it comes to eating. The reason that so many people struggle with eating is that, while it's a necessary act for survival, it is also tied to our upbringing, emotions, and relationships. Perhaps for you, food, in the past, meant a loving gesture from someone in a loving relationship with you. Or maybe not eating was a way for you to protest rules set by a parent or authority figure, by going on a "food strike." Or maybe you experienced food, or lack of it, as a source of punishment.

Through eating awareness we can disarm an emotional or Pavlovian response, by letting go of the triggers and tuning in to our bodies for signals of comfort and discomfort. The shift that must take place is a shift from eating to live, or survive, to nourishing the temple that houses our soul. Eating is a pleasurable, sacred act. It should be respected and revered. In the previous chapter, we discussed dharma. How can you live out your dharma if you're feeling lousy all the time because of the food you're consuming or how you're consuming it? Believing with all your heart that food is medicine will change the way you approach food altogether. You will no longer be imprisoned by the food itself, food commercials, and artificial products on grocery shelves. Instead you'll be looking for ways to optimize your energy level with proper food intake.

Ten Guidelines for Eating Awareness

1. EAT ONLY WHEN YOU'RE HUNGRY. This may seem like a no-brainer, but how many times have you eaten only because you looked at the clock and noticed that it was coffee time, snack time, or lunchtime? A good exercise is to put your hand over your stomach, close your eyes, and feel if there's any undigested food left in there. You might feel a slight sense of fullness. Or you might also feel a little indigestion; or if you burp, you can taste undigested food. That's a good indicator of an undigested meal. Another way to decide if you really need more food is to keep track of when you last put anything in your mouth besides water. For Vata types, two

to four hours should go by before they eat again. Pitta types should wait three to five hours between meals, and Kapha types should wait four to six before eating again.

2. **EAT IN A CALM ENVIRONMENT.** Your body should not be agitated from extreme noise, blaring lights, or a heated debate when you're eating. You also should refrain from watching TV, listening to the radio, browsing the Internet, texting, and talking on the phone. You can't remain aware when you are distracted.

3. **PUT DOWN YOUR FORK BETWEEN BITES.** Enjoyment from eating comes from pacing yourself. You can't enjoy your food if you're shoveling it in. You're not a garbage disposal. I can assure you: no one is going to take your food away from you.

4. **EAT TWO CUPPED HANDFULS OF FOOD AT A MEAL.** You would be surprised how effective portion control is at making it possible for you to lose weight, maintain weight, or feel comfortable after a meal. To measure how much two cupped handfuls is for you, start with a dry substance such as uncooked rice. Fill a bowl with the rice, and set an empty bowl nearby. Using both hands together, scoop up enough rice to fill your hands, and place it in the empty bowl. Do that twice. Then, using a measuring cup, measure the amount of rice you put in the second bowl. Most people will find they've scooped out about two or three cups of rice.

5. **STOP EATING WHEN YOU'RE SATISFIED BUT NOT FULL.** When you're satisfied, you usually sigh once. You look at your plate and say, "That was good." If your plate is still half full, have someone take it away, or put the leftover food in a container, or throw it away instantly.

You may have no clue what "satisfied" feels like because you've always eaten until you're full. But with practice you will regain the ability to detect your body's signals of satisfaction.

6. **DO NOT EAT IF YOU AREN'T ENJOYING YOUR FOOD.** Please, for your health, respect this guideline. I have fallen into the trap of eating bad food, and I imagine you have too. Just because the food is in front of you, you eat it — even if it's poor quality, too greasy, too fatty, or just plain disgusting. Maybe you have a fear of wasting food, or apathy has crept in. Whatever the reason, remember that the energy that comes from the food will be nourishing your body and your cells. If the food isn't appealing to you, your cells won't like it either.

7. **SIT DOWN TO EAT AT A TABLE WITH A PLEASANT SETTING.** Please do not eat while sitting in your car, standing in your kitchen, or walking around a park or mall. Sit down and be mindful of what you're doing. Clear out your eating space. Remove papers, books, computers, mail, and bills before sitting down to your meal. Put some fresh flowers or candles and a nice place mat or tablecloth on the table. Again, it's impossible to extract all the good healing chemicals of a fresh meal if you're staring at a Visa bill for five thousand dollars lying on the table.

8. **DRINK ONLY WATER AT MEALS, IN SMALL AMOUNTS.** Drinking large amounts of anything dilutes the gastric juices and makes digestion difficult for your body. The water should be at room temperature; take only small sips throughout the meal. Any other beverage should be consumed outside of meals.

9. **Do not eat when you're upset.** Eating a pint of Ben and Jerry's Chubby Hubby is not going to heal your relationship with your spouse, and finishing off a cheesecake will not make your mother stop telling you what to do. It's also true that skipping a meal because of an emotional upset will not kill you. You likely have some reserved energy in your body that will make up for that one meal. But eating while upset can create a host of digestive issues and may make you sick. Just sip warm water until you've calmed down or feel genuinely hungry again.

10. **Feel gratitude for the food you have.** Give thanks to the Creator, in whichever way you conceive it, to the cook, to the waitress or waiter, or to anyone else involved in preparing and serving your food. Even if you don't see them directly, have gratitude in your heart. This sense of gratitude will allow the best digestion and assimilation of nutrients possible.

Eating for Your Mind-Body Type

If you do nothing else but apply the Twelve Guidelines for an Ayurvedic Lifestyle Eating Plan and the Ten Guidelines for Eating Awareness, you will see your health improve markedly. But if you'd like to learn how to eat for your mind-body type, be sure to read the following pages, where I outline some simple steps to take.

A dosha-specific diet is the most effective diet to follow when you detect that your body is out of balance or out of sorts. Once you begin getting back in tune with your body, you'll notice when imbalances start to occur. You may first notice a general sense of fatigue. If you're a Vata type, you may notice dry skin, dry eyes, restlessness, trouble sleeping, or more worry than usual. Typical Vata imbalances also include constipation and excess gas. A Pitta type may notice a bit more irritability when going out of balance. She may experience high acidity, acid reflux, or oversensitivity to spicy or sour foods. An out-of-balance Pitta can also experience skin rashes or acne. A Kapha type will eat more than usual and notice some weight gain or feel heavy and lethargic. Nasal congestion, excess mucus, and complacency are all symptoms of an out-of-balance Kapha.

When you go out of balance, the dosha that is specifically out of balance starts to increase in the body. Since you don't need more of what you already have, increasing the dosha will make you feel a sense of discomfort. For example, a Kapha type already has a fair amount of the water and earth elements in his mind-body constitution. Let's suppose that a Kapha has been eating a lot over the holidays (increased earth), has been snowed in and forced to stay indoors for a few days (increased earth and water from the weather and inertia), and has now caught a cold, which causes chest and nasal congestion (increased water). The heaviness of the food, the inertia of remaining indoors, and the increased mucus all cause Kapha to increase in the body. To counteract the increased Kapha, this person would do well to follow a Kapha-type diet to decrease Kapha.

REMEMBER: *You don't need more of what you already have naturally.*

Try a dosha-specific diet for your dominant dosha for three to five days, and notice if you experience improvement. In addition to following the diet, drink a dosha-specific herbal tea in between meals. Remember, you are not eliminating the other tastes; you are increasing the tastes that balance your dosha and reducing the tastes that can aggravate your dosha.

The question on this subject that generally arises is: "If I have two dominant doshas, which diet do I follow?" As a general rule, follow the dosha-specific diet that corresponds to the stronger dosha. However, if you find that your symptoms reflect the second-most dominant dosha, follow that diet instead. For example, if your prakruti is Vata-Pitta, follow a Vata-pacifying or -specific diet. But if you're experiencing acid reflux, loose stools, and your skin is warm to the touch, you have excess Pitta and should follow a Pitta-pacifying diet instead. Another easy way to decide is to take the season into consideration. In Pitta season (summer), for example, follow a Pitta-specific diet. In Vata season (fall–early winter), follow a Vata-specific diet.

It may seem like a great balancing act (no pun intended), and it is. Because of the food we eat, the liquids we drink, the experiences we have, and the emotions we process, we are in constant flux between balance and imbalance. It's not an exact science, however. But now that you're aware of your natural state of being (prakruti) and what it feels like to go out of balance (vikruti), you have the tools to keep the pendulum from swinging too far in one direction or the other.

If we examine the five great elements and the six tastes, we can see how each corresponds to an increase or decrease in the elements in our mind-body constitution:

SPACE (AKASHA): increased by the bitter and astringent tastes.
AIR (VAYU): increased by the bitter, pungent, and astringent tastes.
FIRE (TEJAS): increased by the pungent taste.
WATER (JALA): increased by the salty and sour tastes.
EARTH (PRITHIVI): increased by the sweet taste.

A Vata-Specific Diet

Since Vata is composed of space and air, a Vata diet will contain mainly foods that have a good amount of water and earth (the qualities opposite of space and air). Here's what to do:

INCREASE: sweet, sour, salty
DECREASE: bitter, pungent, astringent

First of all, to counteract the already light and cold Vata dosha, Vata types must eat warm, heavy, oily, and sweet foods. To give some examples, home-cooked foods such as stews, casseroles, pasta dishes, hot apple pie, bread pudding, and hot bread with olive oil are all Vata pacifying. Vata types can eat cold foods, but only in very warm weather. Vatas respond best to cooked vegetables rather than raw; warmed 2 percent or whole milk rather than skim milk; and sweet fruit such as mangoes, ripe bananas, and pears. The three tastes that Vata types should focus on are the sweet, sour, and salty tastes, and Vatas should eat smaller quantities of bitter, pungent, and astringent foods.

A Pitta-Specific Diet

Remember that Pitta is made up of fire and water. Pitta types need to stay cool and reduce some of the water. The best type of foods for Pittas are cooling foods with sweet, bitter, and astringent tastes:

INCREASE: sweet, bitter, astringent
DECREASE: sour, salty, pungent

Unlike Vata types, Pittas do well with salads and colder foods all year long. Pittas can eat raw veggies and beans, lentils, and sprouts. Often Pitta types do best with a vegetarian diet. Since their appetites are good and sometimes ravenous, Pittas need to be careful about not overeating, even when they eat the right foods. To regain balance or remain in balance, a person with a Pitta constitution should steer clear of spicy and greasy foods, minimize red meat intake, and avoid alcohol consumption. A Pitta should also minimize additional salt intake.

A Kapha-Specific Diet

Since Kapha is composed of water and earth, Kapha types need more space and air or lighter qualities. This means they need a diet that is the opposite of a Vata diet:

INCREASE: bitter, pungent, astringent
DECREASE: sweet, sour, salty

Kapha is a cold dosha like Vata, but Kapha types generally do well with raw vegetables and salads as long as they're not ice cold. The bitter, pungent, and astringent tastes help balance Kaphas, who should reduce their consumption of the sweet, sour, and salty tastes. Kapha-type food examples include spicy hummus, lentil soup, stir-fried green vegetables and tofu, leafy green salads, lean fish, vegetable burritos, berry fruit salads, and almonds. Spice should be added whenever possible to jump-start the Kapha metabolism, and small amounts of caffeinated coffee or tea are completely acceptable to help boost a Kapha person's energy level. To rebalance themselves, Kaphas should eat breakfast later in the morning or skip breakfast altogether. Kapha types need two decent-sized meals or one small and two medium-sized meals, with no snacking in between.

Exercise: Your Dosha-Specific Eating Plan

Using the guidelines about dosha-specific eating above, the six tastes list on pages 64–65, and the sample meals on page 66, create a plan for one day's meals according to your dominant dosha. If you are a two-dosha type, you may need a plan for both doshas depending on the season. You will generally eat for your dominant dosha in three seasons and follow the diet for your secondary dosha in the appropriate season for that dosha. The seasons are generally split as follows, but they may vary according to geographical location: Kapha season is late winter to spring, Pitta season is summer, and Vata season is fall to early winter. Make sure you include all six tastes at every meal.

BREAKFAST:
LUNCH:
SNACK:
DINNER:

Feeding the Temple That Houses Your Soul

Ayurveda teaches us that there is energy in everything. This energy, called prana, or vital life force, exists everywhere. It is my wish for you to experience a shift in awareness when it comes to food and feeding your body, mind, and soul. Consider the idea that prana exists not only in your food, water, and drink but also in the energy you put into preparing your food. Have you ever eaten a dish prepared with love? It could be a cake or soup your grandmother always prepared or that homecoming meal your mom makes for you each time you visit her. Doesn't that food taste and feel so much better than when you prepare it?

Eating is a sacred act we all must participate in at least a few times a day. Strive to find the joy in shopping for food, preparing food, and enjoying it. The love, joy, and happiness you feel will bring you the energy in it. When you prepare food for your family, cook with love. On a similar note, the food that nourishes this body that houses your soul should never be referred to as just "calories." You are not simply "filling the tank." You are creating prana. You are creating vital energy, which will give you joy to carry with you throughout your day.

So many of us complain that we don't have energy, that we're tired most of the time. This is where energy starts. Feed your body properly, add mindfulness to your eating, and consider it a sacred act. Then, and only then, will you start to heal the physical body.

Daily Routine and Seasonal Routine: Respecting Nature's Waves

All of nature respects a certain dynamic. There are cycles in nature. The seasons change. There is a cycle of birth, life, death, and rebirth. Deciduous trees and hibernating animals sleep during the winter. The sun rises and sets each day, bringing our planet day and night. Butterflies and birds fly south for the winter and come back in the spring. And if humans don't disrupt it, everything happens according to plan.

As part of nature, we too must respect nature's waves. Our ancestors respected nature's waves, before the advent of electricity, because they were connected to the earth. Now we are disconnected from nature. In the United States, we can shop in stores or online twenty-four hours a day. We can dine or watch TV at any hour. Connected to us by our electronic devices, our jobs, friends, and families make demands on us all the time, anytime. We are "on" continually, unless we force ourselves to take a break. A couple days ago I was at my son's choral concert and was surprised to see not only kids but also adults using their handheld devices during the whole event. What happened to enjoying the moment?

I constantly see clients who say they don't have a moment in the day to themselves. And when I go over their daily routines, I discover that they can, in fact, take time for themselves. With continual activity in our days and nights, it's no wonder anxiety and stress are taking away our health. Ayurveda teaches that we must respect the cycle of rest and activity if we are to enjoy a healthy life. We simply cannot just go, go, go until we drop dead. Where is the enjoyment in going all the time? And what are you trying to get to?

An Ayurvedic Daily Routine

According to Ayurveda, doshas govern not only the seasons but also the daily or circadian rhythm.

The twenty-four-hour clock is divided into six parts:

2:00 to 6:00 AM: Vata time
6:00 to 10:00 AM: Kapha time
10:00 AM to 2:00 PM: Pitta time
2:00 to 6:00 PM: Vata time
6:00 to 10:00 PM: Kapha time
10:00 PM to 2:00 AM: Pitta time

2:00 TO 6:00 AM: VATA TIME

The body is in a hypermetabolic state. Sleep is important during this time because the dream state, which is the most prominent state during this period, cleanses your mind and emotions. Waking up just before six assures you of a more alert feeling in the morning.

6:00 TO 10:00 AM: KAPHA TIME

The body shifts to a hypometabolic state. Waking up late in this Kapha period can leave you with a groggy, heavy feeling all morning. It's best to wake up at the beginning of the Kapha period or earlier and to get started with your day. This is a good time to meditate, do some light yoga such as Sun Salutations (for instructions, see the appendix), and, if you're a Kapha type, do some cardiovascular exercise and strength training. Kaphas can wait until nine thirty or ten to eat breakfast if they have little hunger. Vatas should eat something warm, and Pittas should eat something before they get their day started.

10:00 AM TO 2:00 PM: PITTA TIME

This is the time of day when the digestive fire is at its height. The biggest meal of the day should be eaten between noon and two. Respecting the guidelines for eating awareness, take time to eat away from your desk and other distractions. Sit quietly for five minutes after your meal, and if possible take a ten- or fifteen-minute walk after eating.

2:00 TO 6:00 PM: VATA TIME

During this second Vata period of the day, the body is once again hypermetabolic. If you didn't overeat at lunch, you should feel energetic and mentally active. The end of Vata time is good for meditation, and if you didn't exercise in the morning, now is an optimal time for it.

6:00 TO 10:00 PM: KAPHA TIME

Your body is winding down, preparing for sleep. Eat a light supper, take a short leisurely walk afterward, and do low-key activities. Strive to be in bed close to ten.

10:00 PM TO 2:00 AM: PITTA TIME

Have you ever gotten the munchies late at night? If so, it's because your digestive fire has once again ignited, but this time in order to digest your food and do cell repair. During the second Pitta period, you should be asleep. The expression "beauty sleep" appropriately describes this time. The Pitta fire is destroying damaged cells, repairing others, and regenerating and rejuvenating your body. So the bottom line is, don't eat during the second Pitta time. Toxins will accumulate in your body, because your body will focus on digesting food before removing toxins and repairing cells.

Routine for Optimal Sleep

In my practice, I've found that a large number of my clients have sleep disturbances. For some it's due to stress at home, financial worries, or stress in the workplace. There are several things you can do to naturally sleep soundly at night. Before you turn to sleep medications try these first.

MEDITATE DAILY

As explained in chapter 4, an ideal routine is to meditate twice a day, in the morning and evening, for twenty to thirty minutes. This practice alone has helped 90 percent of my clients who have sleep disturbances.

CREATE A COMFORTABLE SPACE DESIGNED FOR SLEEP

Many sleep experts agree that the bedroom should be reserved for sleep and intimate activities. Remove all clutter from your bedroom. Keep dirty laundry, laundry baskets, bags, and other items out of the vicinity of the bed. TVs and other electronics shouldn't be in the bedroom, because they provide distractions and emit a field of electromagnetic energy. Put your favorite artwork or inspirational quotes, beautiful pictures, flowers, or scented candles in the room.

AVOID CAFFEINE AND ALCOHOL AFTER 4 PM

Sometimes sleep issues are caused simply by drinking coffee, tea, or soft drinks too close to bedtime. Switch to herbal teas or water if you must drink something before bedtime. And if you customarily drink alcohol, then be aware that, according to the National Institutes of Health, even a drink during happy hour can cause wakefulness in the second half of sleep.

Avoid Snacking during the Two or Three Hours before Bedtime

According to an Ayurvedic daily routine, you should eat a light supper about three hours before bedtime. Ideally, you won't be eating anything else until the next day. This recommendation helps to induce sleep when you're ready to rest and helps keep weight gain at bay.

Avoid Mentally Stimulating Activities or Intense Exercise an Hour or Two before Bedtime

Doing your budget or taxes or watching intense psychological thrillers or even the news before bed can engage the mind. Opt to skip the news, leave work or unfinished bills until the next day, and read some inspirational or spiritual literature instead.

Place Aromatherapy Oils on Pillow or Sheets

Certain scents like lavender, vanilla, jasmine, and chamomile can help induce sleep. You can buy ready-made essential-oil sprays or make your own with distilled water. Make sure you're using real essential oils, which are more concentrated and last longer. You can put a couple drops of essential oil on your pillow or sheets or place them on a cotton ball and leave it under your pillow. A low-maintenance solution would be to place a lavender sachet under your pillow in the morning and keep it there until you're ready for sleep.

Journal to Unload the Thoughts of the Day

One of the biggest complaints I get in my practice is: "I can't turn my mind off." Journaling is one of the best ways to clear the mind before bed. It doesn't matter how you do it. You can write about your day or about your thoughts and feelings or even create lists of things you need to do the next day. An enlightening exercise is to write down all the things you are thankful for. There is power in putting things down on paper, and it works to clear the mind for sleep.

Go to Bed at the Same Time Every Night and Wake Up at the Same Time Each Morning

This seems obvious, right? And it does work. Ayurveda recommends being in bed and asleep by 10 or 11 o'clock and waking around 6 in the morning. When you train your body to go to sleep at a certain time, it will expect sleep. The greatest imbalances occur when you have an erratic bedtime and waking time.

Take a Warm Bath or Shower and Massage Yourself with Warm Sesame Oil or Vata Oil

In your bath, you can use the same aromatherapy scents listed earlier in the aromatherapy section. Ayurvedic practice includes a self-administered massage called *abhyanga*. In the evening, an effective massage takes about two minutes. Use a massage-grade sesame oil or a Vata (dosha-specific) oil (the Chopra Center in Carlsbad, California, makes a nice, relaxing Vata oil). Generally, a Vata oil is used as a sleep aid even for the other doshas, since it is calming. Pour about a tablespoon in your palm and start massaging the backs of your ears, easing down to the back of your neck. Then, massage your stomach in a clockwise motion and end with the soles of your feet. This technique can also be used on small children and babies who have a hard time sleeping.

DRINK A CUP OF WARM MILK WITH NUTMEG AND CARDAMOM OR HAVE CHAMOMILE OR VATA TEA

Warm milk has traditionally been used as a sleep inducer, and an Ayurvedic recipe calls for a pinch of nutmeg and cardamom; you can also add a teaspoon of sugar. Equally, chamomile tea is a natural tranquilizer. Vata tea, made from Vata-pacifying herbs and good for all doshas for sleep induction, can also help. Mapi.com sells a nice Vata tea for a reasonable price.

SLEEP WITH THE LIGHTS OFF

This advice may seem like common sense, and it is. But you may be among the large percentage of people who sleep with a certain amount of light on. For the release of the proper amount of hormones, such as melatonin, your body needs darkness. Even a dim light or the flicker of a TV can inhibit the production of this hormone, causing not only sleep disturbances but also depression.

INCLUDE THIRTY MINUTES OF CARDIOVASCULAR EXERCISE IN YOUR DAILY ROUTINE

In the next section, we will discuss physical activity and the ideal types for your dosha. But something as simple as brisk walking can assist you in getting a good night's sleep.

Moving Your Body

Thinking about physical activity is new to the human species. Until about seventy-five years ago, humans naturally engaged in physical activity as a part of daily life. If you lived in the country, you worked on the farm or in a garden; if you lived in a city or the suburbs, you walked everywhere. Simply by performing daily activities, people got the exercise their bodies needed and then some.

In America today and in other industrialized countries around the globe, people need to think about moving their bodies in a way that will keep them healthy. Think about your day and daily routine. Does your current daily routine encourage you to remain sedentary? And for the most part, do you remain inactive?

If you want to live in optimal health, you must move your body in some form of activity. Exercise keeps your muscles strong, removes toxins from the body, and helps with digestion, sleep, hormone production, and more. There is absolutely no replacement for daily activity, and no magic pill that will help.

The Three Components of a Fitness Program

In order to make your exercise regime complete, you must include three components: cardiovascular movement, strength or resistance training, and flexibility training. Many exercise programs combine at least two of these.

Cardio training is probably the most popular because it's the easiest to achieve. You can get your thirty minutes of cardio by doing activities such as walking, running, biking, hiking, dancing, and gardening. Here's the tricky part, though: Everyone has a target heart rate, at which the heart is working at about 70 percent of its capacity. This target zone changes according to your weight and age. In order to benefit fully from your cardio workout, you must sustain this target heart rate for at least twenty minutes. The healthier you are and the older you get, the more difficult it is to achieve this with a walking regime. You may need to do interval training or pick up the pace in any of your activities for your heart rate to stay within your target zone. The best way to know if you're in your target zone is to buy and wear a heart rate monitor. They are relatively inexpensive and worth the investment.

Strength or resistance training is the second component of a complete fitness regime. Use hand weights, weight machines, or your body's own weight for resistance. The older we become, the more muscle mass we lose, so strength training is as essential as cardio.

Flexibility is the third component. To keep us young, healthy, and balanced, we need to include flexibility training.

Ayurveda emphasizes yoga because it has been practiced with success for so long and has a great number of benefits, not only for the physical body but for the emotional and spiritual bodies as well. The word *yoga* is Sanskrit for "to yoke" or "to join together." What we celebrate in yoga is the union of the mind, body, soul, and spirit. One set of poses, in particular, called the Sun Salutations, or Surya Namaskar in Sanskrit, is extremely beneficial. This series of twelve movements exercises every major muscle group in the body and takes care of flexibility and strength training. When sustained for at least twenty minutes, the Sun Salutations can also be considered a healthy cardiovascular practice as well. See the appendix for diagrams of the twelve movements.

Yoga has become popular in the marketplace in the past few years, but let me add a note of caution. Not all yoga instruction is beneficial. At the Ayurvedic Path Yoga studio, we practice a safe form of yoga called hatha yoga. We make sure that students get into and out of poses safely. We teach students to honor their bodies and to abstain from any pose that doesn't feel right. The best yoga practice teaches you to access your inner yogi rather than accept orders that urge you to do poses your body is not ready for.

In addition to yoga, you can do some simple stretches, Pilates, or tai chi.

Moving According to Your Mind-Body Type

While any exercise or activity that moves your body is good, there are certain activities that are ideal for each mind-body type.

VATA TYPES

Being composed of the elements of air and space, Vata types have peaks and valleys of energy. They need an exercise regime that is gentle and creative, one that sparks their interest. Vatas do best with walking, swimming, dance, yoga, aerobics, light jogging, or a sport that is not too strenuous. Also, Vata types need to mix up their routines so they don't get bored. Their vital energy is quickly depleted, so running a marathon may not be good for a Vata type.

PITTA TYPES

These intense individuals are composed mainly of fire and water. Naturally they are attracted to activity, but mostly for the competitive aspect. Pitta types like to win. They have more stamina than Vata types but need to watch the fiery aspect of their personality when playing sports so they don't get too fierce in their competitiveness. Pitta types do especially well when exercising outdoors. They can handle running, jogging, walking, aerobic activity, biking, and hiking; swimming is especially beneficial for Pittas. In my practice, I get a fair amount of Pitta types who like to do hot yoga (yoga practiced in high temperatures). This is counterintuitive for Pitta types, who already have enough fire. Practicing activities in the heat can aggravate Pitta.

KAPHA TYPES

The slowest moving of the three doshas, Kapha is composed of water and earth, so Kaphas need movement in their daily routine. Getting it can be a challenge, since Kapha types are less inclined to move. They need the most rigorous of activities, and it helps if they have a goal, such as training for a 5K run or a marathon. Their solid structure and stamina allows them to handle endurance sports. Kapha types should exercise during morning Kapha time, between six and ten. Engaging in activity at this time will boost their metabolism and keep them more energetic all day. Kaphas can also handle heated yoga fairly well, and it can be good for them. Even meditation for Kaphas can be a moving meditation.

Exercise: Creating Your Physical Movement Plan

Any activity you do should be enjoyable. Following an exercise plan you dislike is not going to bring you the most benefit and will not keep you motivated. Learning a new skill can take time, but if you have fun doing it, it will be far more beneficial in the long run. For example, I've taken up salsa dancing. While it's difficult to learn, it's challenging my brain and my body, I have fun, and it keeps the Vata side of me from getting bored.

Below is a sample physical movement plan; use it as a guide to make your own plan — one that reflects your interests and constitution. Remember to include the three components of a fitness program: cardiovascular, strength/resistance training, and flexibility. If you are mostly Vata, you will need to include variety, maybe changing activities every other day or every third day. Pitta types will need a couple of different activities and perhaps one that will take them outdoors. Kaphas can create a plan and stick to it, since they don't like to deviate from routine. In your plan, include at least five days of activity a week.

A SAMPLE ROUTINE FOR A VATA TYPE

MONDAYS AND WEDNESDAYS: sixty minutes of hatha yoga (for flexibility and strength).

TUESDAYS AND THURSDAYS: walk briskly for forty-five minutes using a heart rate monitor (cardio).

FRIDAYS: go to the gym and do thirty minutes of cardio and thirty minutes of weight training (cardio and strength).

SATURDAYS: go salsa dancing (cardio).

✔ Checklist for Health
Physical Healing

❑ Read over and start applying the Twelve Guidelines for an Ayurvedic Lifestyle Eating Plan.

❑ Go through your kitchen cupboards, refrigerator, and pantry. Purge any food with artificial anything. Toss out foods, including dressings and sauces, that are old or expired or that contain any ingredients such as hydrogenated oils and high-fructose corn syrup.

❏ Start stocking your kitchen with organic items: grains, spices, basic healthy oils, and broths.

❏ Remember, less is more. Eating fresh is more important than buying in bulk. Save money by purchasing smaller amounts of fresh, organic food rather than big packages of food you will likely discard anyway.

❏ Prepare a sample breakfast, lunch, and dinner menu for your Ayurvedic mind-body type.

❏ Read and start applying the Ten Guidelines for Eating Awareness.

❏ Create a reasonable daily routine and post it on your bathroom mirror.

❏ Create a plan for exercise and movement. Start by following it twice a week then add one day of movement per week until you've achieved five days weekly.

CHAPTER FOUR

SPIRITUAL HEALTH

We are not human beings having a spiritual experience.
We are spiritual beings having a human experience.

— PIERRE TEILHARD DE CHARDIN

Ayurveda is a consciousness-based system of health that includes spiritual practices. At my yoga center, I have found that many clients who suffer physical and, more important, emotional symptoms, have neglected to include a spiritual practice in their daily lives. If you are in that category and are not sure how to integrate a spiritual practice, or are hesitant, this section will give you the tools you need in order to begin.

What Defines *Spiritual*?

Defined simply, the word *spiritual* relates to the human spirit or soul beyond the physical or material. The problem with the concept of spirituality is that people either love it or hate it.

Most don't understand what it really means to be spiritual. And others associate spirituality strictly with religion. If we truly are spiritual beings having a human experience, as Teilhard de Chardin proposes, how is it that so few of us actually know what this is about?

I believe the intimate link between the word *spiritual* and the word *religion* has caused mistrust in the concept of spirituality because of the imperfect nature of religion as an institution. Many people I meet state they are spiritual but not religious. Yet upon further conversation I realize that they are, in fact, more religious than spiritual. Even though some people prefer to embrace the concept of spirituality rather than religion, sometimes that's difficult to do. Most of us have been brought up in one religion or another. Religion, like a person's cultural or educational upbringing, becomes ingrained in the fabric of who we are; and no matter what we do to change the course of our thinking or belief system, it remains there, like a faithful friend. And in denying this fact, we often find that this faithful friend becomes more present. So if you were brought up Christian, Muslim, Jewish, Hindu, Buddhist, or something else, just accept it as a part of your upbringing. But it doesn't mean you can't expand upon what you've learned.

Spirituality, on the other hand, while related in some way to religion, is a whole other ball game. I believe that, because spirituality, unlike religion, is difficult to delineate, many fear the subject. The fear may come from our inability to explain it. To paraphrase Dr. Deepak Chopra, "When something happens which we cannot explain, we call it a miracle. But when we discover the reason why, we call it science. Yet, it does not make it less miraculous."

Our knowledge of what is, is extremely limited. If we were to base our thinking, beliefs, and sense of possibility only on what we know, we would be living in a tiny box. And most of us do. It's as if we've moved into a house of one hundred rooms and, instead of exploring or even being aware that we live in such a house, we confine ourselves to four rooms. Of course we can live a decent life in those four rooms, but why not explore the other ninety-six?

It is imperative that, in the process of healing or living a life of wholeness, we expand our view of life and the possibilities contained within it. So, when we define spirituality, we can expand our view beyond religion and, as a result, also have a sense of intuition and experience such things as coincidences, good luck, love, awe, compassion, wonder, and excitement. And when we expand, we feel a sense of connectedness, trust, surrender, and flow. Then we experience the miraculous.

Please understand, it does not matter what religion you adhere to, if any; you can and do live a spiritual life. It also doesn't matter if you believe in a higher being. I've met self-proclaimed atheists who weren't actually atheists at all. Many had been disappointed by their own concept of God, such as when they asked for something that didn't manifest in their lives. Others had been so turned off by religion that they concluded that anything related to a life of God creates violence, chaos, and disharmony. And some, who believe that nothing exists beyond the physical realm or that which can be proved, have opted out the possibility of a higher being. However, most atheists admit there is something else, whether it is called Mother Nature or universal organization. Call life beyond the physical what you will. But a life of healing cannot occur without embracing this part of you.

Embracing Your Spiritual Self

In cultivating your awareness of your spiritual self, it's essential to turn inward to find it. All our lives we have been called to the outside world in everything we do. When we were born, our attachment to our parents or other caregivers gave us what we needed to survive. We looked to those same caregivers, as well as siblings, grandparents, and other family members, to help us form our concept of self and our place in the world. In school, we looked to our teachers and friends for approval and guidance. In every part of our lives — at work, in relationships, and in daily life — we are drawn outside ourselves. How often have you been asked to look inside yourself?

In order to get in touch with our spiritual essence, we must expand our view of what it means to be spiritual. I believe the easiest concept to begin with is intuition. Often we struggle to make decisions, forgetting that the answers we seek are contained within. Have you ever been in a situation where you "felt" danger, although you couldn't quite put your finger on why? Or have you ever met someone and, in an instant, had a sense that this person would be your new best friend? If so, you were homing in on your intuition.

Since the body, mind, soul, and spirit are interconnected, when you begin to connect to this sense you will feel sensations in your body guiding you in the right direction. You will no longer struggle to make decisions. Ask your body if a decision *feels* right, and you will get an answer: either a sinking feeling or a feeling of ease. A successful Japanese businessman was once asked how he became so successful. He answered that he felt his body before making any business transaction, and that the answers his body gave him were never wrong. Heightened intuition leads to spontaneous right action or decision-making, if you follow it. When pondering a decision, close your eyes, place your hand over your belly in the area of your solar plexus, and ask the question. Wait for a sensation in the body. With practice, you will begin to understand your body's signals and become sensitive to what's right for you.

Going from Tunnel Vision to Funnel Vision

Our agreement with reality has been formed over time. As newborns, we embraced infinite possibilities. And then our parents began to tell us what to do or what not to do. Then began the process of turning our expansive view of the world into a constricted view. The process of cultural and social conditioning gives us tunnel vision in all that we do, think, and perceive. Often the conditioning is so strong that we make decisions or think thoughts without knowing why. Have you ever bought something or performed some other action by habit and then said to yourself, "Why am I doing this? I don't even want this." Let's say you have a habit of getting coffee and a donut at ten every morning, but then one day you realize you don't really like donuts. It's just something you've done for years. Awareness is the result of coming to that realization and, the next day, buying a yogurt or a piece of fruit instead. Lack of awareness is knowing you don't like donuts but continuing to buy them because it's what you've always done.

Buying a food item is a trivial example, but we go through this process all the time with decisions big and small. Suppose you've gone to church every Sunday because your parents taught you it was the right thing to do. In this case, you hate your church, wake up in a bad mood on Sunday morning, drag yourself to Mass, put in your time, and head home. Then one Sunday, Mass is canceled because of a snowstorm and you stay home. You snuggle in your favorite chair, take out some inspirational literature, stare in amazement at the snow glistening in the sun, and feel a sense of contentment and connectedness to all that is. You tell me which one of those actions is more expansive. I am not implying that going to church is a bad thing. I am suggesting that listening to your inner voice and honoring it connects you to your spiritual self. Social and cultural conditioning were necessary to get you where you are today. But if you are going to open up the other ninety-six rooms, you need to let go of that conditioning. Letting go may be temporary or permanent. It's a choice. But it becomes conscious choice-making rather than conditioned choice-making. And with conscious choice-making, we're better prepared to live with the consequences of our choices, whether good, bad, or neutral.

Another reason why most people stick to their four rooms is that doing so is familiar and comfortable. Holding on to what we know keeps us in our comfort zone, even if we're not content. The first time you begin to question your choices or thoughts, and then take action in the direction that feels right but different, can be extremely scary. You are stepping into something new and unfamiliar. The voice of past conditioning can be very loud: "You shouldn't do that," "What if…," or better yet, "We've never done it that way; that's not the way it's done." If you hear these conversations in your head, shut them out for now. They are remnants of your past holding you back. You can let them back in when you're ready. Then question them to see if they are true. One false belief that we hold on to when living in fear of moving forward is that there's no going back. As you expand your awareness, you're exploring new horizons. Who says there's no going back? There's no rule stating that once you've left your previous conditioning, you can't go back. You always have that possibility. Let's take the example of going weekly to church: Suppose you decide to skip church for a few weeks and try out your new Sunday ritual. Then, after a month or two, you decide you actually miss going to church, or that it was inspirational for you. Will someone levy a punishment or fine if you go back? I doubt it.

For a brief time, I was a Girl Scout leader for my daughter's troop. The badges earned on their vests are called Try-Its. The girls earned each Try-It when they accomplished three or four items on a list, which proved they had actually tried a new activity. I thought the name and concept were brilliant because they encouraged the girls to try new things without feeling that they had to like them or adopt them permanently into their lives. As adults we need to do the same. Try new things, test the waters, start to expand your vision of reality, and see what works.

Cultivating the Act of Witnessing Awareness

When we stay mired in our thoughts, we usually stay in the realm of past conditioning. Once we begin to witness our thoughts, we can determine whether they are old and outdated or new and evolutionary.

The concept of becoming a witness is simple. In a new environment, you do this all the time. You take in the sights and scenery and listen to the sounds: you notice what's happening all around you. Once we're used to an environment and have assessed or judged a situation, we stop witnessing. We go about our day on autopilot unless something interrupts our pattern. Other terms for witnessing include *noticing* and *observing*. Watch yourself as you go through your day — observe your thoughts, actions, and words. Don't judge yourself, just watch.

The better you become at observing yourself, the easier it will be to pick up on patterns in behavior that are no longer serving you. The first step is noticing. And when you're ready, you can set your intention to change those patterns into ones that will serve you better.

Another tool to cultivate is listening to your internal dialogue. We all have conversations with ourselves, which include phrases we repeat endlessly. Witness your internal dialogue. Notice when you repeat things to yourself. Do you hear negative self-talk? Are you telling yourself things that may be no longer true?

In my classes with Dr. David Simon, he used to explain that there are three gateways between a thought and speaking. Before something slips through your lips, ask yourself these questions: Is it true? Is it necessary? Is it kind? The questions were intended to address dialogue with others, but you can apply them to your inner dialogue too.

Take the first question: Is it true? We repeat things to ourselves for years without regard for their truthfulness. For instance, I grew up with the notion that I couldn't play sports. When I was young I didn't have good hand-eye coordination, especially when it came to sports played with a ball. My automatic response and thought pattern became: "I can't play sports." One day, I realized that this response might not be true. I was asked to join a volleyball game on the beach, and instead of making my usual response, I agreed to play without saying anything. Now instead of repeating a phrase that is not true, I may say, "I'm not especially good at basketball," or, "I'm rusty and need practice." Those statements are true.

Here's another example. I have a client who's single and who has recently lost a lot of weight. She looks fabulous and is naturally beautiful. She said to me, "I can't stop thinking when I'm out in public: 'I'm unapproachable. Guys do not approach me.'" Looking at her, I thought the statement completely absurd. In order for her to make a truthful statement, she needed to shift her inner dialogue to something like: "I'm thin and beautiful. Guys will approach me with ease."

Let's suppose that a statement you're repeating to yourself

is true. But it may not be necessary to repeat it. Maybe you were from a broken home or grew up without knowing your dad or were orphaned at a young age. While these statements may be true, continually repeating them doesn't open up your life to newer possibilities and healing, so let them go.

The third question, "Is it kind?" is probably the most important one. As you begin to notice your internal dialogue, do you notice kindness? Are you kind to yourself? Are you kind to others in your thoughts? If you can answer yes, you are on the right path, regardless of how others perceive you. Start with kindness toward yourself, especially as you begin witnessing your awareness. Wherever you are now in your journey, if you never notice your patterns they can never change.

Exercise: Internal-Dialogue Assessment

As you begin to notice your internal dialogue, write down the phrases that come up most often, either internally or in the things you say about yourself to others.

Phrases I repeat to myself that are positive:

Phrases I repeat to myself that are negative:

Next, turn the negative thoughts or phrases you wrote down into ones that are more positive or are going to serve you better.

EXAMPLE: Turn the negative phrase "I am lazy" into a positive one like this: "I'm learning to make lists and manage my time better each day."

Meditation: Anyone Can Do It

One of the best ways to cultivate the act of witnessing awareness is to practice meditation. Meditation is the quieting of the mind field. It lowers the number of thoughts we have in a day. It brings calm stillness to the mind and body and helps us access our higher, or spiritual, selves.

When taught properly, meditation is fairly easy to do. At the Ayurvedic Path, we practice a mantra-based meditation technique called Primordial Sound Meditation, which is also practiced at the Chopra Center. Another type of mantra-based meditation practice is Transcendental Meditation. In my experience, mantra meditations are among the most successful because the mind is given something to do. You silently repeat a mantra, which is a sound without meaning, and the mantra replaces thought. The nature of the mind is to think thoughts, and if you go into meditation with the intention of stopping thought altogether, it's nearly impossible.

Even if you have no formal training in meditation, you can sit in silence with your eyes closed for a few minutes each day. Find a spot in your home or office where you have few or no distractions, close your eyes, and observe your breath for five minutes. If your mind wanders, bring it back to your breath. Don't try to control your breath; just watch. You may notice that it gets faster, or maybe it falls into a pattern. That's okay; just let it be.

Meditation is beneficial on every level, from physical to emotional and spiritual. To name a few benefits, it lowers blood pressure, normalizes heart rate, increases immune capacity, decreases stress hormones, and improves sleep. The effects of meditation on the body are quite different from those of rest or sleep. You do experience restfulness after meditating, but the benefits are slightly different because the body is in a different state.

Find a meditation teacher in your area to learn how to properly meditate. It can be frustrating to do it on your own. In the appendix, you will find a few websites that might help you locate a meditation teacher or center near you.

Two main reasons why most students who have an interest in meditation don't meditate are that they believe their minds cannot be calmed, and that meditation is a waste of precious time.

Thinking Thousands of Thoughts a Day

When talking with my yoga students about learning meditation, the most frequent excuse I hear is: "I think way too many thoughts. I could never sit still and turn my mind off." In response, I always laugh because that was me before 2007.

The nature of the mind is to think thoughts. It's said that we have anywhere from fifty thousand to sixty thousand thoughts a day. Most of those thoughts are the same ones we had the previous day. Needless to say, the mind is a pretty busy place. If you can relate to having many thoughts, too many thoughts, or even a hundred thousand thoughts a day, know that you are normal. Having thoughts means you are alive. Congratulations!

The practice of meditation helps to lower the number of thoughts, creates new thoughts instead of repetitive ones, and aids in the evolution of thought. Your mind will become calmer. There will be periods of silence in the mind instead of constant chatter. Because of the society we live in, the mind is on hyperdrive. Even as I sit here writing this, I hear the *ping* of my iPhone letting me know I have an email. As I hear the *ping*,

I am tempted to stop writing and check my email. The constant call of numerous means of communication, and other distractions, adds to the chatter. Meditation in your daily routine will slow your mind down, sift through and separate the useless from the useful thoughts, and make your life easier.

In the beginning, when you start meditating, it's not easy. As soon as you sit down and become silent, the mind has all kinds of things to say to you. At this point, an untrained meditator may quit and get up. But if you stick with it, the mind eventually allows you some silence. Before I started my formal meditation practice, I learned guided meditation from a nurse practitioner during my cancer treatment. She taught me to watch my thoughts like an old movie flickering across a screen. While sitting in meditation, you will see a thought arise, transition through your mind space, and — if you do nothing with it — go away. Judging it or asking questions of it will make it stay longer. But if you simply watch it and let it alone, it will drift by. Meditating is much like watching yourself go through daily activity, but instead of watching your activity you will be watching your thoughts.

As I have learned, I am entirely in control of my thoughts. You are the thinker of thoughts, so you have control. The nurse I mentioned earlier told me, when I did my own Internal-Dialogue Assessment exercise (described in the section on witnessing awareness), that if I had a disturbing or upsetting thought I could put flowers around that thought and let it go. Your mental image can be flowers, white light, or whatever else makes you feel good. Don't supply power to negative or disturbing thoughts. You have that choice. Through this observation, you will learn that you are not your thoughts. You are the orchestrator of thoughts.

Meditation is not about stopping thought altogether. Stopping it is virtually impossible. You may experience a pause in thought, which is called slipping into the gap or space in between thoughts, but you won't stop your mind completely. But what we *can* do is use a mantra in meditation as an instrument to replace thought. Typically, mantras have no meaning, and so they do not create associations. In silently repeating a mantra, you replace thought by giving the mind something else to do. One useful mantra is *so hum*. This mantra can be silently repeated with one breath: *so* on the inhalation and *hum* on the exhalation. It's easy to use and can be prolonged with a longer breath to slow down your breathing.

Deciding that you can't meditate because you think too many thoughts is the same as deciding that you can't eat because you're afraid of eating too much. It's ridiculous!

Do Nothing or Do Everything?

Another excuse for not meditating that people frequently make is: "I feel like I'm wasting my time while meditating when I could get so many other things done." I previously used this excuse too — and still do sometimes, even though nothing could be farther from the truth.

Meditation is a connection to everything that is. As you meditate, you plug into universal energy. We live so independently, thinking we can accomplish and achieve everything on our own. We live by mantras such as: "I have so many problems," "I have bills to pay," and "My house is a mess." With this mind-set, we strive never to arrive. We're so busy doing that we don't take time to be, to allow. It's in the allowing that we create open space for whatever it is we desire to come to us.

When you're constantly doing, making lists, accomplishing tasks, going for the goal, how many problems do you encounter?

In that mode I have found that I encounter quite a few. And when you hit these roadblocks, you get angry, frustrated, and anxious. But what if you came across the same problem and let it go instead, trusting that you would find the solution in time? To do this, you would add the problem to your intentions list, sit silently in meditation, and allow the solution to come to you. In this way we solve problems better, more efficiently, with little error. In your doing mode, you probably bulldoze your way through problems and, because of the frustration and anxiety they provoke, make rash decisions that may turn out wrong. Can you remember a time when this happened?

So here is my rationale. Because we connect to universal energy in meditation, our lives become better organized and more efficient, and we waste less time. Decisions become easy. We enjoy life more because we're less worried, nervous, and stressed. The right people simply show up at the right time. Life flows. And when you do encounter another problem, you set an intention to find a solution, you state that intention before you begin meditation, and then you let it go. The universe will handle the details for you.

Wondering How It Works

Honestly, I don't fully understand how a computer works, yet I use one every day. I trust that it will store my information, retrieve that information when I need it, and take me to the Internet daily. I simply trust that it will work. The type of computer I use, MacBook Pro, has been tested by computer experts and used by countless numbers of consumers; and Macs have been around at least since the beginning of home computers.

No one fully understands how and why meditation works, either, but it does. Studies using electrodes have allowed researchers to scan brain waves during meditation, when the body enters a state of calm, wakeful awareness. This relaxed state differs from sleep, according to a joint study on nondirective meditation by researchers from the Norwegian University of Science and Technology and Sydney University in Australia.[1] During meditation, delta waves, the brain activity waves associated with sleep, are decreased, while alpha and theta waves are increased. So, as you meditate, your brain is actually processing information, experiences, and emotions, allowing things to work themselves out.

This may be why, according to a study based on the use of Transcendental Meditation and published in the *International Journal of Neuroscience*, researchers found that the biological ages of meditators were on average five to ten years lower than their chronological ages. Meditators are continually de-stressing.[2] And if you're still not convinced, let me point out that a tool used successfully for thousands of years may have some credibility.

Living a Spiritual Life

You can home in on your intuition, practice witnessing your awareness, watch your thoughts, and meditate or pray. But living a spiritual life also requires practicing right action. Throughout the years, I've collected suggestions from authors and speakers on the subject of spirituality. And while I could discuss many more here, I've narrowed the list down to ten things you can do each day to get in touch with your spiritual self.

1. Practice Gratitude

Every morning, wake up and say thank you. "Thank you for this beautiful day." "Thank you for a new opportunity." Whatever makes you arise from your bed happily, give gratitude for it.

Every time anyone does anything for you, say thank you. Express gratitude in everything you do. When you get caught up in a bad mood, stop and find something to be grateful for. Life is too short to get wrapped up in self-pity, and we receive so many gifts. Be thankful. Give thanks to your creator, however you perceive him or her. We have a tendency to use God as a vending machine. Say thank you instead.

Create a gratitude journal and write in it every day. If nothing else, write, "Thank you for the air I breathe."

2. Have a Namasté Day

I love this exercise, and I encourage all my meditation students to do it. The word *namasté* is a greeting. But the essence of the word is: "I honor the light in you, which is the same as the light in me, and I know we are one." When you say namasté, you are honoring the other person's soul, not her body, mind, position, or social status. And souls don't wear Prada, Gucci, or Louis Vuitton. In other words, in universal consciousness, every one of us is equal.

Pick a day when you will encounter many people, from cashiers to coworkers to family members or friends. Designate that day as your Namasté Day. During the entire day, look directly into the eyes of everyone you encounter and silently bid those people namasté. It takes a brief moment to look into someone's eyes with the intention of honoring her soul, but the rewards are amazing. Afterward, go about your business with that person. But notice what happens. The conversation will take a different turn. She may smile more. You may smile more. The interaction becomes more pleasant, grounded, and surprising. Even if nothing earth-shattering happens the first time, repeat the exercise throughout the day and observe. You will notice a difference at least in how you feel.

3. Immerse Yourself in Nature

We have developed a "box" lifestyle. We live in a box. We get into a moving box to go to our "work" box. Then, we may head to the gym box and back to our home box. You could probably go for days without actually being outdoors for more than a few minutes at a time. This counters our inherent nature — we are mammals, after all. Up until about a hundred years ago, the human race had to spend time outdoors to get food, grow food, and build and maintain shelter. Even though we've created these boxes, we remain intimately linked to nature and need to experience it to stay healthy. Allow the sun to shine on your face. Saunter barefoot through the grass. Take a walk outdoors daily. Sit and have your morning coffee outside. Find a way to immerse yourself in nature daily.

4. Experience Wonder and Awe

Instead of going through life with blinders on, wrapped up in all you have to do, stop and embrace the simple but miraculous world around you. Take moments in the day to watch birds fly, observe a child at play, catch a sunset, or take a new route to work and notice something new.

We tend to program ourselves to do the same things with the same routine, and we lose our sense of wonder. Notice that small children are amazed at most everything. The world is such an astonishing place, and there are many new things to discover and old things to observe.

5. Take Time to Laugh Each Day

This may seem self-evident, but truly laughter can heal you. According to research by Robin Dunbar and his colleagues, evolutionary psychologists at Oxford University, laughter produces endorphins and natural pain-relieving chemicals — which are equally produced by physical activity.[3]

Start by smiling often. Smile as you answer the phone; smile at the lady at the coffeehouse who gives you your morning coffee. Find something to laugh about. Life should be a joyful experience. Laugh especially at yourself. It helps not to take yourself so seriously. Motivational speaker and author Leo Buscaglia said, "Laughter is like changing a baby's diaper. It doesn't solve anything, but it sure improves the situation."

6. Give Someone Your Full Attention Each Day

Have you ever been conversing with a friend, only to have her look down, check her phone, and text someone while you were talking? If we are to live in the present moment and connect with our higher selves and others, it's important to practice staying immersed in the present. Give one person today your full attention. Tomorrow, increase it to two people. Notice when you get distracted by devices while you are with other people.

7. Hug Often and Touch Often

Human touch is certainly one of the most fundamental aspects of health, wellness, and happiness. It saddens me to think that so many people spend each day without being touched by another person. Hug your neighbors, your friends, your children, and your lover. Find opportunities to touch someone's hand, shoulder, or face. In this society we have become so afraid of touch — because of potential lawsuits or accusations of sexual misconduct — that we have disconnected ourselves from this fundamental human need. My youngest son, a second grader at the time and only seven years old, was told by his teacher that he could not hug his best friend because there was a "no touching policy" in school. My thought was: "What is this world coming to that children are taught in school not to hug their friends?"

8. Perform Random Acts of Kindness

Each day, find something nice to do for someone at random. You could buy a colleague a cup of coffee. Offer to take a friend out for dinner. It could be a small thing that costs nothing, such as letting someone into your lane while driving. Kindness is all about connection and reaching outside yourself and your own problems. Next time you're feeling self-pity or sadness, go out and do something for someone else.

9. Forgive, Let Go, and Move On

Forgiveness is the fragrance that the violet sheds
on the heel that has crushed it.

— MARK TWAIN

Life is too short to hold on to grievances. When someone hurts you and you fail to forgive, the poison in that arrow penetrates you, not the other. Chances are, the other person has forgotten what happened. And when you hold on to the pain, it keeps you from moving forward. Forgiveness is internal. You can inform the person or persons who hurt you that you forgive them, but it's not necessary for your own healing.

Once you've forgiven someone in your heart, let go of the grievance completely. Don't allow the memory to haunt you further. If it's something you've held on to for a while, it's already taken up a portion of your life. The last part of the process is moving on. People grow and change, as do relationships.

When you allow yourself to forgive, even *you* change. And forward is the direction you must go for healing and growth to occur.

10. Love Like There's No Tomorrow

Being love is absolutely the best way to embrace your spiritual self. In subsequent chapters we will focus more on emotions, relationships, and your past. But for now, suffice it to say that being loving is the best way you can be. More of your true self comes out in love than in any other way. Observe yourself showing and giving love. By far, it is the most important thing you will ever do.

✔ Checklist for Health
Spiritual Healing

❏ Explore your own definition of the word *spiritual*.

❏ Listen to your intuition. Feel signals in your body when you have decisions to make.

❏ Pay attention to the choices you make, and decide whether they are based on social conditioning and habit or on conscious choices.

❏ Notice your internal dialogue. Write down your positive internal dialogue, and create a plan to turn around negative internal dialogue.

❏ Learn meditation and practice it twice a day for twenty to thirty minutes each time.

❏ Practice living a spiritual life by experiencing gratitude and by giving.

CHAPTER FIVE

EMOTIONAL HEALTH

*If your emotional abilities aren't in hand, if you don't have
self-awareness, if you are not able to manage your distressing
emotions, if you can't have empathy and have effective relationships,
then no matter how smart you are, you are not going to get very far.*

— DANIEL GOLEMAN

One of my teachers once said, "You can do all the meditation you want, but if you don't do emotional clearing, it's all
for nothing."

There is an undeniable connection between physical and
emotional health. They are so closely linked that sometimes
it's difficult to see the distinction between the two. Mothers
have this intuitive sense of the connection, such as when, for
example, a little one suddenly develops a "stomachache" every
morning before school. Mom will ask questions, only to find
out a classmate has been bullying him. The physical symptoms
manifest on school mornings, when the child fears seeing the
bully at school. I once heard that there are more heart attacks
in middle-aged men at nine on Monday morning than any

other time. Is that a coincidence? Or is it the dread of a hated job that causes the heart attack at that particular time?

Ayurvedic medicine looks for this mind-body connection. A practitioner will certainly look at the physical being, observing the patient for any signs of imbalance, but then will ask the patient what's going on in his or her life. Everyone has a story. I see many clients suffering from chronic diseases such as Lyme disease, fibromyalgia, and generalized pain. Especially in these clients, I always look for the emotional component. And there is always an emotional component. Either there's a recent divorce, death in the family, trouble with a child or parent, or financial strife that's led to excessive stress. To reemphasize this point: you cannot heal if you don't heal your emotions.

My best friend's mother was diagnosed at age sixty with an aggressive form of ovarian cancer. She was told she had a 30 percent chance of survival. But the doctor told her family that her chances were actually lower than that, because he had rarely seen anyone live through the treatment let alone survive and tell the story. She not only beat the odds but also had almost made it to her five-year mark when she was again diagnosed with cancer — this time an aggressive lymphoma — and was once again given a 30 percent chance of beating her cancer. When she finished her treatment and went into remission, I asked her why she thought she had gotten cancer again. She responded, "I had hate and resentment I was holding on to toward my husband. I worked through the anger, let it go, and forgave him for anything he did. It was only then that I was able to heal." She is alive and well today at age seventy-eight and has outlived her husband, with whom, she said, she had a second honeymoon period. Clearly, she saw and experienced the power of emotional healing.

Do You Run Your Emotions,
or Do Your Emotions Run You?

Just as you have some control over your thoughts, you also have a certain amount of control over your emotions. Sometimes we become overwhelmed with emotions, but even then we are in control of what happens when we feel them. Too many of us believe we are victims of our emotions. Men blame their anger on their aggressive nature. Women blame their crankiness on PMS. In reality, we are evolved creatures, and we can choose not to react like a conditioned bundle of nerves. When it comes to what we let into our bodies and what we don't, we have access to a higher intelligence. Certainly, we are hardwired differently from each other when it comes to our propensity to react a certain way. Vata types have a tendency toward worry and nervousness. Pitta types get more irritable, judgmental, and angry. Kapha types get possessive, clingy, sad, and depressed. This natural inclination toward one reaction or another doesn't mean you won't experience a whole spectrum of emotions, but you will become aware that you've started to react in a particular manner. You can either choose to go there or choose another way of dealing with the emotion. In this way, you no longer remain a prisoner of your emotions.

There will be times, though, when you can't control your emotions, and appropriately so. Upon hearing the news that a loved one has died or had an accident, you may be overcome with sadness, and that's the appropriate response. But if you find you continue to respond with sadness to thoughts of that event for years after the initial news, you probably have some emotional clearing to do.

Or suppose you are predominately a Pitta type and you find yourself getting angry and irritated more often than usual. You can use self-observation to figure out why your Pitta is out of balance and work on rebalancing it through diet, outdoor exercise, taking in some fresh air, or maybe venting to a good friend. Once you regain control, you can go to the root of why you've been getting angry so often.

As a Vata type, I tend toward worry. I keep myself in check when I find I'm worrying too much: I call a good friend, drink some Vata tea, and get a good night's rest. Once I'm back in balance, I'm better able to assess whether the emotions had any validity at all.

Have you ever found yourself overreacting, then realized that it was useless to even react? Then, you're left picking up the pieces of your reaction, often with embarrassment. I once saw a poster for an anti-child-abuse campaign that stated, "Count from 10 backwards before you think about hitting your child." It's often that deep breath, counting, or changing scenery that prevents us from reacting with emotion.

With practice, you'll be able to treat your emotions as thoughts and realize that emotions come and go. If we don't give too much weight to them, they subside with time. If we process them properly, they have less power over us when they come back.

Tools for Establishing a Healthy Emotional Life

According to Ayurveda, we not only process food and drink, but we process emotions and experiences as well. When we don't process our food properly, our body accumulates toxins, develops free radicals, and creates cellular instability leading to diseases such as cancer or heart disease. When we fail to properly process our emotions and experiences, we create toxins of another sort. Emotional toxins come out as anxiety, depression, sadness, hopelessness, anger, rage, impatience, or guilt.

Have you ever eaten a meal while arguing with someone and found that the meal did not sit well in your stomach afterward? Your argument created emotional toxins; this manifested as indigestion from a meal.

Over time, we accumulate these emotional toxins, and if we don't clear them regularly they manifest as physical symptoms and, ultimately, disease. The following sections offer some tools, including regular emotional clearing, that you can use to keep your emotions in check.

Meditate Daily

The effects of meditation on emotional health are extremely helpful. When you begin to meditate regularly, emotions that have accumulated for years tend to come up. Know that this is normal. Look at it as an emotional detox. When you start exercising after a period of inertia, the body begins to rid itself of toxins. Meditation does this to your emotional body, so it's not to be feared. In the beginning you may experience sadness or may cry. You might think about someone who left your life long ago. Whatever your experience, let it come up, because it represents unresolved emotions from your past. If you become overwhelmed during your meditation, it's okay to stop and write down your thoughts and feelings. The more you've been stuffing your feelings, the more will come up. Celebrate it! You're getting healthier.

Another positive effect of meditation on your emotional health is your reactivity to events, emotions, and experiences. When you meditate, you enter a state of calm awareness. After your meditation, you tend to remain in this state for a while. This nonreactive state remains intact when something happens, and so you tend to have a delayed reaction or a reaction that differs from what's normal for you. Often meditators tell of letting things just slide off their backs instead of reacting to them. I like to explain that it's like taking a step back from the situation as if you were an observer. This happens without your even trying, as a result of your meditation practice.

Take Responsibility for What You Are Feeling

Taking responsibility for your feelings is, by far, the most important level you can reach in emotional health. Long ago, I read a brilliant book called *Emotional Intelligence* by Daniel Goleman. The premise of the book is that, if your emotional intelligence is low, it does not matter what your intelligence quotient is. Instinctively we know this when we see people behave obnoxiously, or out of control, in public. However, our society puts greater emphasis on measurable intelligence and gauges it through testing, grades, degrees, and so on. From the time we are put in school, we are constantly compared and evaluated according to what we know. Little emphasis is placed on our emotions, how we manage our feelings and events, and how we treat others and ourselves. In the real world, success depends more on emotional health than IQ. Let me give you an example. If a CEO of a company consistently gets angry with employees, he will not be able to successfully lead a company. In relationships, partners who take responsibility for their feelings, instead of constantly blaming the other when things go awry, are more successful at problem solving and relationship building.

One thing you must realize is that no one put your feelings there in the first place. You put them there. We can interpret events, circumstances, words, and exchanges in many different ways. If we respond negatively, it's because we have preset our notions or ideas about how things should be. The other person or persons that we interact with are not responsible for our preset notions.

Don't get me wrong. There is absolutely nothing wrong with having any type of feeling about a given situation. Feelings are a normal part of our human existence. It's what we do with those feelings that matters.

Let's suppose you try on a new dress for a party. You ask your partner's advice about the dress. He hesitates then says, "Let's see you in this black dress over here." Inside, you negatively interpret the comment as: "He doesn't like the dress" or "He thinks I don't look good" or "He thinks I'm fat." Whichever the negative interpretation, you might feel rejection, disappointment, sadness, anger, or frustration at the comment. Whatever it is you're feeling, take ownership of it. When we take ownership of a feeling, the feeling has a tendency to dissipate.

So let's suppose that in this example you are disappointed because you suspect your partner is indicating you are fat. But your partner didn't mention anything about fat; he simply suggested trying on another dress. Many situations that provoke strong feelings are based on assumptions rather than confirmed fact. But even if your feelings are completely justified, remember that they are yours.

Deal with the Emotion as It Occurs

Ignoring emotions is like ignoring a persistent toddler. They will bother you until they get what they want. We tend to perceive our emotions as notions in our head, and to perceive feelings as emotions experienced in the body — that is, we perceive emotions intellectually but also physically, as if they took two different forms. Examples of emotions are love, joy, anger, frustration, or disappointment. We may feel the emotion of love, in the body, as a lightness in the heart, an airy head, or butterflies in the stomach. And in the body, we may feel anger as a "hot" head, a churning stomach, or tense muscles.

After taking responsibility for a feeling you are experiencing, identify the emotion: happiness, sadness, love, anger, hate, frustration, urgency, impatience, or desperation. Once you identify the emotion, feel where you sense it in your body. Sometimes when you are frustrated, and you link it to your body, you realize you're hungry and the growling stomach, not the situation, has made you frustrated. Or perhaps you react negatively to a coworker, but when you place your hand on your head to assimilate the emotion, you come to the conclusion that your anger is due to an email you read minutes before.

A great way to identify an emotion and link it to your body is to ask yourself some questions:

- What am I feeling?
- Where am I feeling it in my body?
- Why do I think I'm reacting this way?
- Have I reacted this way to a similar situation before?
- Do I see the possibility to react differently?

The entire time, remain nonjudgmental with yourself. You are simply gathering clues to your reaction.

Then pay attention to your body. You might want to breathe deeply a few times into the area where your body is experiencing discomfort in response to the feeling. As you breathe, notice that the discomfort starts to dissipate in response to your attention.

Be a Conscious Choice-Maker

Once you are aware of your feelings, you can choose whether you wish to stay with them. You may believe you have no choice but to feel them. But in fact, the choice is yours and always has been. We are used to reacting like a conditioned bundle of nerves, and so we think we have no choice other than to react in the same way we've always reacted. However, nothing is farther from the truth. Let's take the example of the dress. If you reacted with frustration because you thought your partner was saying you are fat, that was just one reaction of many. You could have interpreted his reaction in one of these ways: "Maybe he just prefers the color black" or "Maybe he wants a couple of options to choose from, and then he'll give me his opinion." Both options are pretty reaction-neutral. Don't you agree?

Let's suppose you are driving to work and someone cuts right in front of you with no warning. What would your initial emotional reaction be? Many people would get angry or upset and wonder how someone could be so inconsiderate. But what if you said to yourself, "Hey, maybe that person is late for a meeting" or "Maybe that person just received some bad news" or even "Maybe that person just needs to get somewhere quickly to use the bathroom." Are any of these scenarios possible? Have you ever been in a similar situation, where you were rushed and you unintentionally cut someone off?

As you can see, a given stimulus or situation can create any emotional reaction you choose. If you resist interpreting it, or if you entertain several different interpretations, not knowing which one is actually accurate, you can choose calmness, curiosity, and freedom from less useful reactions.

But let's assume that a situation does provoke a strong emotional reaction in you. Suppose you invite a friend to a movie you really want to see, and your friend is late so you miss the beginning. This particular friend has been late in the past. You stuff down your feelings of disappointment, anger, frustration, or even rage as you see your friend approach, and you say, "Oh, that's okay. We've only missed a few minutes." A reaction such as this does not necessarily make you a conscious choice-maker, because you are experiencing negative feelings and are negating them rather than expressing them to your friend in a healthy manner. Rest assured, they will creep up at a later time. Your ways of feeling and expressing are not in sync. In order to sync them up, you might tell your friend: "You are a dear friend and I love you. But when you are not on time I feel frustrated because I need you to respect my time. In the future, would you mind planning on leaving home fifteen minutes earlier in order to be on time?" This method, called conscious communication by Dr. Marshall Rosenberg in his book *Nonviolent Communication: A Language of Life*, is a means to process our emotions in a healthy way.

Be Process Oriented Rather Than Goal Oriented

Growth takes time. We work hard on our educations, at our jobs, and at being parents and friends. Rarely are we coached on how to work with our emotions. Just like anything else you need to work on, creating a healthy emotional life takes time. You will reach higher aspects of yourself through practice and trial and error. Whatever your age, you've been developing emotional-response habits for that long. Don't expect instant results. As you practice meditation and cultivate your ability to witness your awareness, you will begin to watch yourself, your emotions, and your reactions to situations and others. By becoming aware of your emotional reactions, you begin to notice what you'd like to change. As you observe, remain aware of your desire to change. Notice how each day is different. Be mindful of your triggers. For example, if you are a Pitta type and you haven't had lunch and it's two in the afternoon, your emotional trigger is likely due to hunger. Or if you're a Vata type and it's been cold and windy all day, your reaction is probably a result of physical discomfort. People close to us can also be triggered by their own experiences. You may notice that certain people in your life know how to irritate you. They are pressing emotional triggers in you. When you notice your reactions, write them down and create a plan to eventually change your trigger reaction. Be honest with yourself. If a loved one or friend points out something that has triggered an emotional reaction in you, then instead of getting angry or upset, look inside to see if it's true.

Celebrate each time you honor your desire for change. Enjoy the process of watching yourself grow emotionally.

Emotional Clearing for Each Dosha

Here's a quick guide to rebalancing your emotional body according to your dosha.

Vata Types

Vata types are prone to nervousness and worry, and they need to be mindful of this tendency. Since Vata types are composed of a higher proportion of space and air, they must keep themselves grounded. When you find yourself worrying, make sure your diet is balanced and you're getting enough sleep. Go to bed, and awaken, at the same time each day. Eat warm foods and avoid dry foods. Create a schedule for yourself and try to stick to it. When a situation, job, relationship, or experience starts to get uncomfortable, rather than changing it right away, try staying with it and ride the waves. Create stability in your life and you'll notice that worry subsides. Write down two or three inspirational phrases that you can read or say aloud to yourself when you're too nervous or are worrying too much. A common phrase that seems to work with worry is: "This too shall pass." Another one might be: "Let go and let God." Whatever your phrases, say them often to yourself until they become second nature.

Vata types are able to process their emotions through creativity and creative expression. Writing may be a great way for a Vata to work through a problem and do some emotional clearing. Keep a journal by your bedside table and write about experiences you would like to clear from your mind and body. Letter writing can be helpful whether or not you share the letter. Painting a picture may be another creative outlet for emotional clearing. Movement, too, tends to come naturally for Vata types. Processing emotions through dance — turning on loud music and dancing your emotions away — or pulling out a pair of ice skates and gliding to emotional healing may be just what the Ayurvedic doctor ordered.

Pitta Types

An out-of-balance Pitta tends toward criticism, impatience, judgment, anger, and control. If your mind-body type is Pitta, you've probably noticed these traits in yourself or you've been told you have them. Often, it's a Pitta type's search for perfection that makes him critical. Remind yourself that no one is perfect. Also, a Pitta often takes himself too seriously. Learn to laugh at yourself when you find you're getting too serious. Life is too short to hold on to things that don't really matter. Instead of blaming others when things don't seem to go your way, take a look at how you've contributed to the situation. And if you haven't contributed, then learn from it and move on, or maybe vow to take a more active role next time. Your remedy will be lightheartedness. Learn to attach humor to a situation, although not at another's expense. When you find yourself getting too fiery, take time to cool down. Watch a comedy show or a funny movie, then turn back to the situation or emotion and see if it's lighter.

Your emotional fire can take over your body as well. Look for the signs of acid reflux, heartburn, skin rashes, acne, or loose stool. These are indications that you're allowing your Pitta to go out of balance. If you feel the heat in your stomach, place your hand over it and see what emotions are there. Thoughts are intimately linked to emotions, so as your hand rests on your stomach and you tune in to the related emotions, notice what thoughts come up. Perhaps you've had a recent experience that caused some turmoil and you are angry. The sensation in your stomach (translating as a symptom such as acid reflux), the feeling of anger, and the experience that made you angry are all intertwined. Understanding the symptoms tied to the emotions and to the experiences that caused them can help you learn to communicate those emotions and take responsibility for what you are feeling. As a Pitta type, you have a tendency either to place the blame on the other person when in conversation or to start criticizing. It's best to recognize when this is happening so you can take note of it. Remember, you are not a prisoner to your past reactions. You can choose new ones in the present.

As for emotional clearing, Pitta types thrive best in nature. Going for long hikes in the mountains or along streams, or biking on trails, is great for Pittas. While Pitta types enjoy sports and competition, these are probably not optimal for clearing emotions, since Pittas can get too emotional while being competitive. Going for a long swim at a nice easy pace will help a Pitta type stay cool while sifting through emotions internally. While gazing at a beautiful sunset or admiring the beauty of the earth, bring to mind your recent emotions or the ones you wish to clear. You will find that kinder, gentler solutions will appear to you in those moments. While fire can burn, it also brings warmth and light. Choose the aspect of yourself that brings light, warmth, and passion to others. Create a few inspirational phrases, or write down a few quotes, to keep you humble, cool, and calm when you find yourself spinning out of control emotionally. Here are a couple of quotes to help guide you: "Blessed are the meek: for they shall inherit the earth" (Matthew 5:5), and, by Victor Hugo, "Laughter is the sun that drives winter from the human face."

Kapha Types

Being composed of water and earth, Kapha types can easily fall to the heaviness of their dosha. When out of balance, a Kapha can gain weight quickly, which can in and of itself cause emotional upset. When Kapha types are emotional, they tend to withdraw and become depressed. Inertia can take over, and then all they want to do is sit on the couch. In relationships, Kapha types can get clingy or possessive. The upside is that, because Kapha types are stable people, it takes a lot to upset them emotionally. A Kapha may take many emotional blows before she withdraws completely.

If your principal mind-body type is Kapha, pay attention to complacency. When you find your healthy eating habits falling by the wayside, and you're constantly craving sweets or fatty foods, ask yourself what is happening emotionally. If you've maintained a consistent exercise program or have been going out for daily walks, and you have suddenly stopped your routine, figure out what event occurred just before you stopped. Since a Kapha enjoys the stability of routine, you may have noticed that stopping one usually happens for a reason. Maybe you had a really bad day at work. Or maybe you had an argument with a loved one that remained unresolved. Something is causing you to compromise your healthy habits and is making you more prone to inertia.

As you realize the source of your emotional imbalance, devise a quick plan of action to keep yourself moving. A great form of movement for Kapha types is a walking meditation. While you ponder your situation or set of emotional reactions, walk as long as it takes to move through it. As a Kapha type, know that you will withdraw when things get too tough. Learning how to deal with feelings instantly, instead of stuffing them down and letting the problems stack up, will help keep you balanced. When you are able to process your emotions, reward yourself with something other than a food celebration. Get a massage, or go with a friend to get your nails done. ~~Or if you're a guy,~~ you may want to get a new pair of sports shoes or tickets to an event.

Exercise: Your Emotional Healing Plan

Since we all have triggers, be observant of yours and create a plan to stop emotions from getting out of hand. With a plan, you can process your emotions when they happen and then move on. Take a moment and write down your plan now, by completing the following prompts.

- Three things I notice occurring in my body when I'm emotionally upset:
  EXAMPLES: "I clench my teeth" or "I get a headache."
  1.
  2.
  3.

- Three typical emotional reactions I have to my triggers:

  EXAMPLES: "I eat sugar" or "I start yelling" or "I jump to conclusions about what the other person is thinking or feeling."
  1.
  2.
  3.

- Three feelings I typically feel when I am emotionally upset:

  EXAMPLES: anger, fear, anxiety, depression, guilt, frustration, sadness, rage, irritation.
  1.
  2.
  3.

- Three situations or people that I know can upset me:

  EXAMPLES: "When someone arrives late" or "When the house gets too messy" or "My brother [or sister, spouse, or parent, and so on]."
  1.
  2.
  3.

Now, commit, to yourself, to remain in control of your emotions. You are not a prisoner of your emotions or your past reactions. You have a choice to act and react differently from now on. You are not a conditioned bundle of nerves. There is an infinite number of choices that you can make in any situation. Some potential situations:

- When I notice my body getting tense with emotion, I will:
  EXAMPLES: "breathe slowly," "count to ten," "close my eyes and feel it," "take a short walk," or "meditate."

- When I am triggered into an emotional reaction, instead of engaging in a destructive behavior, I will choose to:
  EXAMPLES: "ask questions instead of jumping to accusations" or "give the other person the benefit of the doubt" or "create a positive story in my head about what *could* be going on."

- My negative feelings about a situation can be turned around with a change in perspective, such as:
  EXAMPLES: "fear can be turned into inquiry" or "sadness can be turned into gratitude or self-love."

- The situations or people who normally can upset me now cause me joy and wonder because I have an infinite number of potential responses to choose from, such as:
  EXAMPLES: "I make a commitment to myself to leave if a friend is continually late, rather than get

upset" or "I will make a list of all the good things my mom [or dad, sister, brother, spouse, or friend] does for me and focus on the gifts in our relationship."

• When I handle my emotions effectively and in a timely manner, I will reward myself by:
  EXAMPLES: "buying myself flowers" or "eating one Godiva chocolate" or "adding money to my vacation savings jar" or "going to get a massage."

Commit to reading Your Emotional Healing Plan daily until it becomes a part of your inner dialogue.

✔ Checklist for Health
Emotional Healing

❑ Explore your normal reactions to see if they are in sync with your Ayurvedic mind-body type.
❑ Determine whether you will control your emotions or allow them to control you.
❑ Practice taking responsibility for your feelings daily.
❑ Complete Your Emotional Healing Plan.

CHAPTER SIX

HEALING YOUR PAST

The past does not equal the future.

— ANTHONY ROBBINS

At times you may wonder why you can't move forward in life. Your intentions are good: you plan to grow, heal, and advance in the direction of your hopes and dreams. But it may seem that something is holding you back. When this happens, it can help to look at unresolved issues of the past. All of us have past experiences that were less than pleasant. But it is our interpretations and impressions of what happened, and why it happened, that can cause us to remain stuck. In this spoke of the wheel, we will explore how to overcome our past and grow beyond it.

What Is Your Story?

Everyone has a story. Our story is our past. We might repeat this story only to ourselves, to others, or both. Often this story weighs us down like a lead cloak, preventing us from moving forward in life. And if it doesn't do that, it at least slows us down sometimes. We use our story as an excuse not to take risks or change our path. We use our story to get sympathy or pity. At times, we use our story as a mask so we don't have to reveal our true self to others.

So what is your story?

It may be simple or long. It may take into account other people or just one person. The story takes the form of a diagnosis, a single experience, or a repeated experience. At all times, your story makes you a victim.

Here are some examples of stories people tell:

- I was abused as a child.
- I was abandoned.
- We were poor.
- My father left when I was eight years old.
- I'm a cancer survivor.
- I come from a broken home.
- I'm a single mother/father.
- I'm a diabetic.
- I suffer from depression.
- I was not given the same opportunities as my brother/ sister.
- I am a middle child.
- My father was an alcoholic.
- My parents were immigrants.
- My parents were married but hated each other.
- I was the "smart" one.
- At school, I was considered a nerd.
- I am fat.

Exercise: The Stories from Your Past

What story or stories do you repeat to yourself and others? Think about and write down at *least* two stories.

How do you feel after writing down your story (or stories)? Better? The same? Do you feel as if your story is familiar to you, like an old friend? Does your story feel empowering?

I will bet your story feels familiar and may feel good. It may even feel safe. But I will also bet it feels disempowering. Your story has been a way to hide from who you really are. It has been keeping you in a holding pattern, preventing you from moving forward. In a sense, your story is an excuse you have made to yourself to not achieve, not take care of yourself, and not live your dharma, or purpose. Now I'm going to ask you to do something radical. Take the pen, pencil, or other writing utensil you used to write your story (or stories) and cross it out. Cross out your story completely. You do not need it in order to succeed in life. You do not need it to move forward in the direction you are moving. It's in your past. Even if part of your story is still occurring in the present, by crossing it out you set your intention to let it go.

Let me explain why this is so important. Though part of your story has some truth to it, another part of it is a lie. Let me repeat, your story, although true, has a grain of untruth to it, so it's not valid. Let's suppose your story is: "I am fat." You could even expand it a bit: "I've been fat a long time" or "I've always been fat."

Yes, your body may be fat. But is that who you are? Have you always been fat? Really? When you were born, for the first few days of your life, were you fat? Was there ever a time in your life when you weren't fat? Even for a day? Is it serving you well to repeat "I am fat" in order to change it?

Instead, change your story to a phrase like: "I am on a path to get healthy and lose weight." Even if you are not sure how to achieve this, but you desire it, you are on the path, right? Is that a more accurate statement? Does it empower you more than "I am fat"?

Let's take another story: "I was abandoned."

Again, this is a partial truth. If you are here today, reading this book, someone raised you. It may not have been your biological parents but someone stepped up to the plate. Perhaps it was your grandmother, an aunt, a stepparent, a foster parent, a neighbor. Someone took the role of parent and helped you become who you are today. Changing perspective helps to change the story and empower you. The story "I was abandoned" can become: "My parents, who were not able to care for me, let my grandmother raise me because they loved me so much."

Exercise: Your New Reality

Now that you've crossed out the old stories, write yourself at least two new stories.

Your story has become so deeply ingrained that it may take some time before you are able to change it completely. Each time you think of the old story, switch to the new one. Remember, while the old story may have had some truth, so does the new story. It's a matter of choice. Shift your focus to the new one in order to move forward.

Understanding Why You Have a Past

The past is tricky. Some of us have a smooth past, and others a difficult one. It's hard to understand the explanation behind what we endured to get to where we are today. If you had a rocky past, you may have come to think that life is unfair. If you had a smooth past, you may wonder what is to come. In Vedanta, the knowledge that Ayurveda derives from, our past not only is our past in this lifetime but also is an accumulation of lifetimes. Whatever you choose to believe, your past and all its lessons got you to where you are today. Have you ever been in the midst of hardship and wondered, "Why in the world am I going through this?" and then found later on that it made sense? There is a bigger picture in the grand scheme of things. Sometimes we receive an answer to the question "Why?" and sometimes we don't.

An expression in Vedanta tells us, "Life flows between the banks of pain and pleasure. We bump into both sides, but we must not get stuck on one side for too long." In the West, we have the expression "This too shall pass," which indicates more or less the same thing. In our hearts, we understand that life is, in fact, like a river. We will always have the dichotomy of good and bad, rich and poor, hardship and ease. When we experience an event, the lesson is not only to witness it but also to gain what it has to teach us. The practice of meditation brings about the ability to witness our awareness. And our intellect will allow us to get the lesson and move on.

In the section on emotional healing, we focused on taking responsibility for our feelings and actions. In learning lessons from past events, taking responsibility is extremely helpful. Often, those who have difficulty moving on after events stay rooted in a victim state of mind, or *victim consciousness*. And if as you read this you're saying to yourself, "Well, I never do that. I don't stay in victim consciousness," guess again. We all do it at one time or another.

Let me provide an example. Have you ever received a speeding ticket? After recovering from shock at the cost of the ticket, you begin to explain to others what happened. Do you tell them something like: "I was going faster than the speed limit, which is against the law. A police officer noticed how fast I was going, pulled me over, and gave me a speeding ticket, which, in the end, I know I deserved because I was breaking the law." Have you ever heard *anyone* say that?

What we usually say or hear is: "It was a speed trap" or "All the other cars were going fast, so I needed to keep up with traffic" or "It was the end of the month, and that cop needed to meet his quota." And those are the nice things we say. But what about: "Those pigs are just on a power trip. Why aren't they out catching criminals instead of picking on poor, law-abiding citizens who are just going ten miles over the speed limit while all those drug dealers and child molesters are running loose?"

Most of us pick victim consciousness because it makes us look like the hero and the other person like the bad guy. But what does it do to our psyche? It keeps us rooted in the past. It becomes a part of our story; we hold on to it, and it keeps us from moving on. Ultimately, we are responsible for all our actions and reactions. It doesn't matter if we did something consciously or unconsciously. If you get this one lesson, you won't believe the personal growth that will occur.

"I am responsible for all my actions and reactions." This is a mantra you can repeat to yourself daily to help you heal from your past. "Now, what if," you might ask, "I did experience an event that I wasn't directly responsible for?"

Let's suppose you were on the receiving end of child abuse, spouse abuse, rape, or another form of violence. I am not suggesting you are responsible for such events. It is obvious that in such an instance you were a victim. But the key word here is *were*. The event happened, however tragic or unfortunate it may have been. And some events are painful enough to take a long time to heal. You are not responsible for those events, but you are responsible for your interpretation of how they affect your present and future. There are stories of survivors of the Holocaust or other instances of genocide, and of mothers of murdered children, who forgave their perpetrators. I've never had anything that tragic happen, and I'm not going to pretend I could easily forgive people who committed such crimes. But those who do have gotten the lesson and moved on.

It doesn't matter what happened in your past. What is it doing to your present and your future?

Finding the Lesson and Moving On

Life gives us tests and lessons. That is clear. What you do with those tests and lessons is your choice. In school, if you take the test, understand the lesson, and score high, you can move on to the next level. Life is the same way. Have you ever discovered a weakness in yourself and found that the same lessons keep popping up as a result of that weakness? Well, it's because you haven't gotten the lesson yet. When you finally get the lesson, the universe will say, "Now's the time to move on." And do you know what that will provide? More lessons! But here's the fun part: once you realize this, you can enjoy it.

The recurring theme in my life is patience. All my life I've struggled with impatience. My mother's repeated words of advice, "Patience is a virtue," kept me frustrated well into adulthood. And my impatience has bitten me in the butt, so to speak. I've burned bridges, missed opportunities, and lost money owing to impatience. Slowly, but surely, I'm getting the lesson. It's taken me over forty years but I am learning to step back and allow things to unfold naturally, rather than forcing things to happen. Now that I'm aware of this life lesson, I get to choose. If I find myself being impatient, I can choose patience.

It goes back to being a choice-maker with an infinite number of options.

Let's say your recurring theme is abusive relationships. Starting with a family member, then a spouse or boss at work, and then others, you've had a stream of abusive relationships. How do you find the lessons in this? Ask yourself these questions:

1. What are these relationships trying to teach me?
2. What do I need to assert verbally or nonverbally to become stronger?
3. How do I step out of the victim role and into an empowered role?
4. What do I need to learn about my patterns of behavior that attract this type of relationship?
5. What am I gaining by remaining in an abusive relationship (or in more than one)?

Again, you are not responsible for having endured abuse in an abusive relationship, but you are responsible for your present and future. By answering empowering questions and setting your intention to move on from the past, you will help yourself receive the lesson. Your recurring theme may not be abuse. It may be poverty, failure, or addiction. It could be procrastination or difficulty with love. Whatever it is, find the recurring theme of your past.

To heal the damage from your past, sometimes it's as easy as making a decision like: "I will no longer allow myself to be in abusive relationships" or "What happened in my past will not decide my future." Other times, healing is a lengthier process that requires professional help. But if professional help is coupled with meditation, self-awareness, taking responsibility, and conscious choice-making, the process of moving forward goes much faster.

The Seven Main Chakras:
Opening Blocked Energy

Regardless of our capacity to heal our past, there is always residue from past impressions. This residue lives in our cells and tissues in the form of toxins. But it also remains in our energy body, the aspect of the self that gives us vital force or vital energy. In Sanskrit, this energy is called prana. Each and every one of us has energy centers in the body called chakras. The word *chakra* means "wheel." There are seven main chakras, and their locations range from the base of the spine all the way up to the crown of the head. If the concept of a chakra, or energy center, is too abstract for you, think of it as an anatomical region that also possesses aspects of your emotions, experiences, personality, and spirit.

An easy example of this is your heart. The heart is the anatomical region, and the emotion most often linked to the heart is love. The experience of love is linked to your heart along with all of your past. Your personal aspect of the heart and love is the way you express love, and the spiritual association of the heart can be anything from self-love to love of a higher being.

To heal from the past and become healthy in the present, and to remain that way in the future, examine the chakras and discover where you're holding on to blocked energy. This can point you in the direction of healing.

When I worked through my experience with thyroid cancer, I was determined to find all the reasons why I had allowed the cancer to occur. Instinctively, I knew the road to healing included the belief that I had brought this to my life, which empowered me to take it out of my life. At twenty-eight I told myself, "I am learning the lesson that thyroid cancer is providing for me so I never have to get cancer again." Through my journey to self-discovery, I learned about the seven main chakras. The thyroid is situated in the fifth chakra, or the chakra of verbal expression.

Once I learned this, I explored internally what I had been doing that kept me from expressing myself fully or, in other words, what had blocked the chakra. And in looking back beyond the thyroid cancer in my health history, I realized that, throughout my entire life, all my ailments had begun in the throat. As a child I'd constantly had strep throat or tonsillitis. When I was seventeen, I was diagnosed with mononucleosis and my throat partially closed as a result of an abscess, which had to be opened surgically. The message was clear: I needed to resolve my throat chakra issues. Expressing my authentic self verbally to loved ones had always been a challenge. However, I didn't recognize it until the moment I gained knowledge about the chakras. I had to go through the difficult task of confronting my fears then and expressing myself to loved ones authentically. Discovering the source of the blockage was liberating. And while it took me some time to honor that part of me, I believe ailments of the throat will never return, now that I've healed the fifth chakra.

When I was in college, I studied Erik Erikson's stages of child psychological development. The premise of his theory is that a child must pass through a certain stage of development at a given age, and if he succeeds, the next step in development will lead him to social and psychological success. The hierarchy of the seven main chakras is similar to psychological development.

Among the seven chakras, three are devoted to the physical; the fourth is the link between matter, or the physical, and spirit; and the last three are spiritual in nature. If you open and align the first three chakras successfully, you will gain greater access to the higher chakras. It is also possible to remain stuck in the first, second, or third chakra and never move to the higher chakras. If you resolve blockages in your chakras, you will gain greater intuition, health, love, happiness, and bliss.

When working to unblock the chakras, it helps to first meditate for about fifteen minutes; then, with your eyes still closed, place your awareness on each of the chakras for about three to five minutes. Your body will let you know where the blockages are located. You will feel either a sense of openness, a neutral state, or a sense of closed energy. In an open chakra, you will feel energy flowing freely, almost as if air could circulate throughout the area of the chakra. When a chakra has a neutral feeling, neither open nor closed, you might feel energy but not exactly free-flowing energy. Since our bodies are in flux between balance and imbalance, a neutral feeling doesn't necessarily indicate a blockage; it may simply be a momentary state. For example, if you just had a meal and you focus on the solar plexus chakra, you might feel movement but not a completely open chakra, since there's food in the stomach. A closed feeling would be a sensation of something solid, such as a lump in your throat when you're upset.

If you detect a neutral or closed sensation in a chakra, keep your awareness there and see if you experience anything related to that chakra. A memory may come to mind, or a symptom you experienced in the past may manifest in the body. Keep a notebook handy while doing this exercise and jot down anything that comes to mind or that you feel in your body. If a lot of memories or sensations are present that relate to a specific chakra, focus your awareness on this chakra a few times a day for the next few days. By maintaining an intention to open the chakra, you will find that you receive guidance on what you need to do to release the energy there. Continue to take notes on what comes up in your meditation practice and in daily activity.

You can use tools to help you open your chakras if necessary. Visualization of the color of each chakra, chanting mantras for the chakra, and wearing gems that correspond to the blocked chakra can be useful. Yoga poses corresponding to each of the chakras, and of course *pranayama* (yogic breathing techniques) and meditation, all aid in chakra opening.

When imagining the area of each chakra, envision it as a thick wheel of swirling energy going from the front of the body through to the back of the body. If you were standing, this "wheel" would be parallel to the floor.

The Root Chakra: Muladhara

This chakra encompasses the base of the spine, the perineum, and the first three vertebrae. The earth element dominates the root chakra, which represents security, stability, basic needs, and trust. When the root chakra is aligned, you feel a sense of security and certainty that your basic physical and psychological needs will be met. An unbalanced root chakra leads to a feeling of being ungrounded, uncertain, and mistrustful. The period when the root chakra builds its foundation is birth to age seven.

When examining your past, look at areas where you might have developed blockages in the root chakra. Things like the death of immediate family members early in life, divorce, loss of a parent's job, relocating frequently, financial loss, or poverty can lead to imbalances in the root chakra. Anytime our foundation is shaken, we create an imbalance in the base chakra.

Possible causes of root chakra imbalance also include obesity, hemorrhoids, constipation, sciatica, degenerative arthritis, anorexia nervosa, knee troubles, greed, violent behavior, fear, anxiety, and insecurity.

The color that corresponds to the muladhara chakra is red, and the mantra sound is *lam*. The gemstones that correspond to the root chakra are ruby and garnet. Any grounding yoga poses are good for the root chakra. *Padmasana* (lotus flexion), knee-to-chest pose, lizard pose, and *sivasana* (relaxation pose) all can open and align this first chakra.

The Creative and Sexual Chakra: Svadhisthana

The second chakra governs our creative and sexual energy. Its location encompasses an area reaching from above the pubic bone to below the navel, and it includes the sacral plexus. Water is the element of the second chakra, which includes the bodily fluids of circulation, urination, elimination, sexuality, and reproduction. *Svadhisthana* is used for expansion. Creative energy is expansion, whether for reproduction or creation of something else new. Expansion leads to growth, and stunted creativity leads to decay. From the second chakra, desire, emotions, and pleasure flow like water. The instinct to nurture is grounded in the second chakra. A healthy second chakra brings us a healthy sex life with our beloved, healthy sexual function, regular menstrual cycles for women, satisfaction in work and play, and creative hobbies. A blocked second chakra can lead to sexual dysfunction; uterine, bladder, or kidney trouble; diseases of the sex organs; addictions; jealousy; envy; or pessimism. We develop the second chakra between the ages of eight and fourteen.

The color of the second chakra is orange, and the mantra sound is *vam*. Coral is its gemstone. Yoga poses that help open and align the second chakra include flowing movements like pelvic rocks, hip swaying, reclining butterfly pose, bound angle pose, and cobra pose. Practicing deep diaphragmatic breathing can help bring energy to the lower abdomen and the second chakra as you consciously expand and contract the belly.

The Solar Plexus Chakra: Manipura

Manipura is considered the dwelling place of the self. Through the third chakra we portray our self to the outside world. This is the chakra of personal power and will. Imagine a large circle around the navel and extending up to the breastbone, and this encompasses the solar plexus chakra. As its name suggests, fire dominates the solar plexus chakra, which is necessary for digestion and assimilation of nutrients in the body. The fire element provides us with the "get up and go" required to perform our work. The solar plexus is also the seat of the ego, which can help or hinder us in life. When aligned, we perform actions of selfless service. An out-of-balance third chakra will cause us to become obsessed with gaining power over others. A blocked third chakra can lead to metabolic disorders such as diabetes, hypoglycemia, and acid reflux and ulcers. We develop the third chakra between ages fourteen to twenty-one.

The color of the manipura chakra is bright yellow like the sun. In fact, the word *manipura* means lustrous gem. The mantra sound is *ram*. The gemstones for the third chakra are amber and topaz. Third-chakra yogic breathing includes the *bhastrika* breath, or the "breath of fire," and *kapalabati*, or the "skull-shining breath." Yoga poses to help open and align the third chakra include the boat pose (*navasana*), bow pose, plank pose with deep breathing, and inclined plane.

The Heart Chakra: Anahata

We've arrived at the center of the seven chakras. There are three below and three above. The heart chakra is where matter and spirit meet. The *anahata* chakra is our source of love, compassion, understanding, empathy, giving, and gratitude. The fourth chakra encompasses the heart, thymus gland, lungs, arms, and hands. The air element rules the heart chakra. Love felt through this chakra is a genuine type of love that goes beyond the sexual attraction of the second chakra and the desire and drive of the third chakra. In the heart, the air element gives us lightheartedness, laughter, weightlessness, and freedom. Ailments of the fourth chakra can manifest as asthma, high blood pressure, heart disease, and lung disease. Another imbalance of the heart chakra occurs when the well-intended giver of love, compassion, devotion, and healing depletes his or her energy without refilling with self-love and self-healing. We develop the fourth chakra between the ages of twenty-one and twenty-eight.

The color of the fourth chakra is green. The mantra sound is *yum*. The gemstones are emerald and rose quartz. Yoga poses that help to open and align the heart chakra include the standing bow pose, camel pose, cow face pose, and fish pose.

The Throat Chakra: Vishuddha

The fifth chakra is the first on the spiritual plane through which we truly transcend our physical limitations. Through communication and verbal expression, we can be present where we are not present physically. Communication via telephone, video, Internet, or audio recordings allows us to transcend space and be in one place while our body is in another place. For example, I can attend a video conference in Tokyo, seeing the attendees and giving my input, while sitting comfortably at my home in Virginia.

Sound, vibration, self-expression, and all forms of communication are encompassed by the fifth chakra. The element corresponding to the fifth chakra is akasha, or space. Sound travels through space. Like akasha, the vastness of communication is infinite.

When the *vishuddha* chakra is open and aligned, we feel we're able to effectively communicate our needs, desires, and ideas. Our connection to others through verbal expression breaks down barriers and provides expansion beyond the personal self.

If the fifth chakra is blocked, we feel a sense of frustration and disconnect, and we're unable to communicate our needs effectively. The anatomical region of the throat chakra includes the thyroid, parathyroid, neck, and shoulders. Physical ailments of this chakra can include sore throat, stiff neck, colds, thyroid problems, or hearing problems. We develop the fifth chakra between the ages of twenty-eight and thirty-five.

The color that corresponds to the vishuddha chakra is bright blue. The mantra sound is *hum*. The gemstone is turquoise. The *ujjayi* yogic breathing technique, which is done with a partially constricted throat and is accompanied by a subtle sound, can help open and align the throat. Yoga poses for the fifth chakra include the plow, shoulder stand, bridge pose, neck rolls and circles, and knee-to-ear pose (a plow pose with bent knees positioned beside the ears).

The Sixth Chakra: Ajna

The sixth chakra is located between the eyebrows and is called the third-eye chakra or the center of intuition. The third-eye chakra encompasses the pineal gland and the eyes. According to Vedanta, the physical eyes see the past and present and the third eye sees the future. The *ajna* chakra brings us clarity, clairvoyance, and spirituality, enabling us to transcend our dualistic nature. Those able to open their third-eye chakra have a glow or a light surrounding their bodies. An out-of-balance ajna chakra can bring about headaches, hallucinations, nightmares, difficulty concentrating, poor memory, eye problems, or difficulty visualizing. We develop the sixth chakra between the ages of thirty-six and forty-two.

The color for the sixth chakra is indigo. The mantra sound is *sham*. The gemstones are lapis lazuli and quartz. Eye exercises are helpful for aligning the sixth chakra. Alternate nostril breathing, or *nadi shodhana*, is a great pranayama and can open the ajna chakra. Yoga poses to help open and align the sixth chakra include the dolphin pose, child's pose supported by pressing the forehead to a block or the floor, and eagle's pose.

The Seventh Chakra: Sahaswara

The seventh chakra, located at the crown of the head, is called the thousand-petal lotus. It is our source of enlightenment and spiritual connection to our higher selves, others, and ultimately the divine. It is at the level of awareness of this chakra that we realize we are not separate from our source but united. Unconditional love flows from our being. The oneness we experience can never again be divided. This is the highest state of attainment in our human existence. The *sahaswara* chakra encompasses the pituitary gland, the cerebral cortex, and the central nervous system. An out-of-balance seventh chakra may bring depression, alienation, confusion, boredom, apathy, spiritual superiority, or loss of memory. We develop the seventh chakra between the ages of forty-three and forty-nine.

The colors are violet and white. The mantra sound is *om*. The gemstones are amethyst and diamond. Meditation is the ultimate practice for opening the crown chakra. Yoga poses that place a focus on the crown of the head, such as the headstand, handstand, and forward folds with the head placed on the floor, help open and align the seventh chakra.

Let Go of Your Past
by Taking Three Lessons to the Future

The past is a guide, a road map that will show you the way to your destiny. Extract from it what you will, and discard that which you no longer need. Deciding to let go is as easy as making a decision. Feel the freedom that arises as you decide to move on. Change the stories you tell yourself and others so you can reshape the path of your future.

From the work we've done together on your story and the blockages in your chakras, what lessons have you learned? What is it about your story that you wish to change? You are the playwright of your life, and you get to write the script. Isn't that exciting?

From your stories and blocked chakras, draw three lessons you wish to take with you into your future. These are lessons you've learned and don't wish to repeat. You've gotten the message from these three lessons, and you are moving on. Some examples: "I no longer need to feed myself unhealthy food to feel whole. I am whole just as I am." "My parents did their best to raise me. I am my own person now who takes full responsibility for her decisions." "I orchestrate my own destiny."

Exercise: Your Three Lessons to
Take to Your Fulfilling Future

1.

2.

3.

✔ Checklist for Health

Healing Your Past

❑ Write down your story as it is today.

❑ Create your new story and write it down.

❑ Explore the lessons of your past and how they formed who you are today.

❑ Go through your chakras and note which ones seem blocked.

❑ Create and write down three lessons to take from your past and into your fulfilling future.

CHAPTER SEVEN

RELATIONSHIP HEALTH

Love is life. And if you miss love, you miss life.

— LEO BUSCAGLIA

True health, growth, and healing come when we have meaningful relationships with others. Too many people are lonely in today's world, and as Mother Teresa so eloquently remarked, "The greatest disease in the West today is not TB or leprosy; it is being unwanted, unloved, and uncared for. We can cure physical diseases with medicine, but the only cure for loneliness, despair, and hopelessness is love."[1] Humans are by nature social beings. We are not meant to be alone. The way to grow into the best version of yourself is through the mirror of relationship.

Relationship starts with the self — getting to know, loving, and accepting yourself at the deepest level. It's the realization that you are not your body, your mind, or your thoughts but something much grander. You are a piece of the greater picture, and your role here, in this parenthesis in time, is important. This discovery is about loving who you are, exactly where you are, because you are, in your essence, a piece of God, or universal spirit. Your spiritual essence is perfect because the source who created you is perfect. When you find this self-love, which is not selfish or self-indulging but giving, you are able to radiate love to all those around you.

It astounds me that, while we are usually able to offer patience, kindness, and love to those in our lives who are experiencing difficulties, when it comes to ourselves and our own insecurities or troubles we are often harsh. To others, we show support and lend a listening ear; we offer them sympathy and kind words. My advice is that you become your own best friend as well. Be patient and kind to yourself. Learn to love your imperfect body and any other flaws you perceive in yourself. Loving them does not mean you don't wish to change some things. You may want to change a behavior that has been weighing you down and preventing you from living a more fulfilling life. But the beginning of your journey starts with self-acceptance and self-love.

More than a year ago, I came out of a relationship with a man I loved very much. Ultimately, this person was not good for me, and even though I loved him, I realized that being with him hindered my growth. One source of pain for me was that, while I loved him, all of him, with all his shortcomings, he was not able to love me the same way. The lesson I learned as we broke up was that he was able to love me only as much as he loved himself. He couldn't possibly give me more love than he had. I could neither blame him for this nor be angry about it.

No one can give more than they have inside. That is why you must start first with self-love.

Furthermore, you cannot love for two in a relationship. Love in a relationship is a dynamic exchange between giver and receiver. The exchange of love will not always be equal. There will be times when you need to either give or receive more. But if you find that you are constantly giving, and love is not given back to you, you will be left empty and devoid of energy. Some people have difficulty receiving love. They find giving is easier. In a relationship, you need to allow the other person the gift of giving to you and seeing you accept it with open arms. Inversely, if you believe the other person continuously owes you something, whether affection, attention, gifts, or acknowledgment, you may need to work on increasing your self-love.

In Ayurveda, relationship is of utmost importance. The life category *kama* (desire and marriage) is one of four important categories in life. The other three are *artha* (wealth), *dharma* (life's purpose), and *moksha* (liberation).

Whether or not you are in an intimate relationship with a significant other, seeking a relationship, or not planning on having one, know that relationship affects us on all levels. We are social animals. Unfortunately, we have built our Western world around the concept of self-sufficiency, which has isolated us. From telecommuting to work, to checking out our own groceries with an electronic scanner, we have taken the human element out of daily life. Think about it: if you wanted to, you could probably go through the day or several days without ever directly interacting with another human being. You can order your food and clothes online. You can pump your own gasoline, drive your own car, send out emails instead of making phone calls, and do your finances without ever setting foot in a bank. Need I go on?

I remember when the state installed automatic scanners on the toll road and I no longer needed to stop and pay the toll. I was a little sad for the missed interaction with the toll-booth employees. It's no wonder that the sale of prescription medication for depression and anxiety is at an all-time high. Our need for self-sufficiency has isolated us and made us completely independent of other humans. But we are by nature social. That hasn't changed. After all, it was discovered not so long ago, in the early 1960s, that infants in orphanages who were not held, caressed, and cuddled, but who received proper nutrition, died. We can change the circumstances, events, and conveniences in daily living, but we cannot change how we are hardwired, hence the intense feelings of isolation and depression that many experience.

A great step toward self-love is recognizing this fact.

We Are Social Beings Meant to Be in Relationships with Others

I understand that some do not want an intimate relationship in the sense of kama, which entails the desire to marry and start a family. But relationships with family members, friends, acquaintances, work colleagues, and neighbors are more important to our health than you may think. How often have you gone to a neighbor's house to *borrow a cup of sugar* in the past year? Do you even know your neighbor? Chances are you've bought a year's supply of sugar at Costco or Sam's Club, and bugs might get to it before you run out. In the West, it has become so easy to live without others that we have to make an even greater effort to include friends and family. And it is essential to do so if we are to attain a balanced life.

Life Is Not Balanced
without Healthy and Loving Relationships

Marital relationships were once the cornerstone of family life, which was the core of social structure in society. From the microcosm of a solid family structure — which included the husband, wife, children, grandparents, aunts, uncles, and cousins — came the macrocosm of neighborhoods, cities, and counties. I remember being a young kid in the 1970s. If I misbehaved and the neighbor on the next block witnessed it, my mother heard about it even before I got home. As daily living has become less centered on family life in the past couple of decades, the social structure of interconnectedness and interdependence has also degenerated. A prime example of this is the changed role of women in society in the past fifty years.

Women are, more than ever, financially independent. This is a blessing and a curse. Just sixty years ago or less, a wife depended on her husband for financial security. While this was a hindrance in the case of an abusive marriage, it also helped keep the relationship together through thick and thin. Today, a woman dissatisfied in marriage or a relationship can bail when she's uncomfortable. The same goes for a man. If he's not worried that she'll be out on the street if he leaves, he's more likely to let the relationship go when the going gets tough. Culturally, relationship breakups are completely acceptable. So where is the glue that holds relationships together?

I am not suggesting that you settle for a lackluster relationship. Part of healing is the expansion of love, compassion, and understanding. Being in a relationship entails embracing the ebb and flow. It's more challenging now than ever to establish stable, lasting, and fulfilling relationships. With the age of immediacy in communication, we expect more of our loved ones. With the facility of communicating with others outside the relationship, infidelity is easier than ever. Not to mention that the lines between being faithful and being unfaithful are thin and fuzzy.

An Ayurvedic understanding of relationship starts with self-awareness and self-love. When you take care of yourself and your physical, emotional, and spiritual needs, you have energy and patience to dedicate to others. Awareness of your own shortcomings and limitations allows you to go easy on your loved ones and their limitations. Recognizing what you need in a relationship enables you to let loved ones know what you need.

In this chapter I focus on romantic relationships, since those seem to be challenging for most. Guidance on communication skills offered here can, however, be applied to any relationship. Humans are universal. We all have the same needs and similar desires, and we deal with the same emotions. And if you haven't yet read the chapter on emotional health (chapter 5), please go back and read it before processing relationship health.

Before we begin, take a moment to reflect on where you are in your relationship, if you have one. Are you currently in a relationship? Are you searching for one? Are you recovering from a recent breakup or divorce? Have you decided to go solo for the moment and discover more about yourself? Wherever you are in regard to relationship is where you are supposed to be. Accept where you are at the moment. If you've read the previous chapter and are working on healing your past, you know that the past is history. Consider the present in relation to your vision for your future.

I was married for a long time. My husband and I met when we were twenty years old, and we casually dated in college. When I became pregnant with my daughter, we decided to do the right thing (according to his and my upbringing) and get married. We were together for a total of fifteen years and had two other beautiful children as well. We had many challenges along the way, but in the end I knew my personal growth with him was stunted. It was a painful decision, but I knew that divorce was best for both of us, because he wasn't able to grow either.

Then I entered into a relationship with a man I fell in love with, but our ideology, morals, and religious upbringing didn't match. We stayed together four years and got engaged, which we celebrated with a huge party. He moved in with me and lived there for a year before things got very bad. He moved out, and I knew right there and then that it was probably best that we hadn't let our relationship drag on any further. After those two experiences, though, I felt defeated. My children had seen me fail in two relationships. For the first few months after the breakup, I was embarrassed and felt I had lost the relationship game. After a lot of soul searching, meditation, reading about relationships, and a seminar on healing the heart, I realized that all relationships are here to teach us something about ourselves. All relationships are valuable, and not all are meant to last.

Let me reiterate: All relationships are here to teach us something about ourselves.

The desperate search for "the one" became much easier when I made a new agreement with reality. I no longer pressured myself to find the perfect relationship with the perfect man that would last the perfect amount of time. Once I stopped pressuring myself, I did find the perfect man for me. He literally walked right into my life and we mutually fell in love straight-away. Do I know how long it will last? I have absolutely no idea, but I know I cherish him and the relationship each and every day. We remind each other how much we love each other several times a day. We let go of the little things that don't matter.

I've told my story to allow you to keep one thing in mind: Where you are is where you are supposed to be.

Do not blame yourself for past failures. If you're in a relationship that is less than what you would like it to be, I will show you how to improve it. If you're searching for a relationship, you will become ready to receive it. And if you're taking time for you right now, read this anyway. It will help your relationships with family and friends.

My mother gave me a great piece of advice when I was very young: "Michelle, make sure you are a whole person before you enter into a relationship with another person." I'm not sure how well I followed the advice, but it's sound. All our work here on living an Ayurvedic lifestyle is meant to enable our return to wholeness. We are returning to wholeness of mind, body, soul, and spirit, which in turn will take us to oneness.

Often a person enters into a relationship to fill a void. That person then becomes a leech, draining energy from the other and eventually suffocating the relationship. Real love comes from wanting it, from desire, and less from need. Certainly, we all have needs, and some of those needs are fulfilled only in a romantic relationship. But if you look to your significant other to fulfill most or all of your needs, you are going to have a problem in that relationship. It's best to enter a relationship from a position of strength, when your strength is at the opti-mal level for you. Searching for a relationship when you've just come out of one doesn't permit this to happen. Other examples of inopportune times: when you are changing or losing a job, times of financial difficulty, when you are in the midst of a court or custody battle, or when you are undergoing therapy. If you are in a relationship and looking to improve it, choose a time when things are in a lull, when nothing major is going on. A time when you have a new baby, or are moving, or have just had an illness or death in the family wouldn't be optimal for working on a relationship.

Twelve Traits of Healthy Relationships

One thing is certain: all relationships have ups and downs. In healthy relationships, however, there are also constants. I've compiled a list of twelve traits of healthy relationships, which I've gleaned from reading many books on relationships, from counseling clients during Ayurvedic consultations, from studying those in successful relationships, and from my own experiences. Those in healthy relationships do the following:

1. Love Each Other Unconditionally

Dr. Leo Buscaglia, expert on love and relationships, wrote in his book titled *Love* that a true relationship filled with love has this one ingredient: unconditional love. According to Dr. Buscaglia, you must love your beloved with open arms. This means your loved one can come and go as he or she pleases and must never feel suffocated, possessed, or coerced into staying with you. Remember the adage that says you must set the one you love free, and that if your love is true your loved one will come back to you?

Unconditional love means you love your beloved when he's fat, thin, ugly, beautiful, nasty, or kind. Think of the love we typically have for our children. Why shouldn't this type of love be applied to our significant other?

2. Accept Each Other for Who They Are

Acceptance goes hand in hand with unconditional love and is a universal human need. We all need to be accepted. Acceptance doesn't mean there is no room for improvement. It does mean that today, when you think about your beloved, you accept exactly where he or she is in life. Everyone's journey is completely different, and you may be on one path while your beloved is on another. If there's a habit or behavior that you need to change, or that you'd like your significant other to change, the change, once accepted, comes from a place of love, safety, security, and acceptance.

3. Don't Sweat the Small Stuff

Frankly, this trait should probably be number one. Many a relationship has ended because of the constant nitpicking that happens in relationships. The nitpicking grates away at the love until there is none left. Unfortunately, many young couples don't learn this until it's too late. The ability to stop sweating the small stuff typically comes with maturity and experience. If you are young, let me save you some time: pay attention to your attitude in relationships rather than the things that don't really matter. Save your energy for discussions of bigger matters, such as finances, children, family, spiritual practice, morals, values, and intimacy.

4. Touch Each Other Often

We all understand that passion is intense in the beginning of a relationship, but the touch you give and experience early on must continue if the relationship is to be successful. People in healthy relationships experience all kinds of touch, from a brush on the face, a squeeze on the shoulder, to hugs, kisses, passionate kisses, and frequent lovemaking. In the chapter on physical health, I emphasized the importance of physical touch. Our skin represents 10 percent of our total body weight. There are more sense receptors on the skin than any other part of the body. The release of growth hormones and healing chemicals is stimulated through touch more than any other sense.

5. Create Memories Together and Cherish Them

I've heard this referred to as *gushing*. Whenever you find yourself in an argumentative pattern with your loved one, start gushing about all the great times you've had together. Create a "remember when" conversation. After reminiscing about all the wonderful memories, start making plans to create more.

6. Understand That Men and Women Have Different Needs and Honor Them

Let's face it: men and women are not the same. The sooner you recognize it, the easier it will be for you to grow in a relationship. A wonderful book that helped me in my marriage is called *His Needs, Her Needs*, by Dr. Willard Harley. It's a Christian-based book, but even if you're not Christian you'll find that the advice is solid. Dr. Harley has counseled thousands of couples, and his findings are the same in every case. The premise of the book is that men and women have distinctly different needs. Once we recognize, learn, and honor these needs, we open ourselves up to a fantastic and fulfilling relationship. One example of a man's need is for his wife or girlfriend to be physically attractive. An example of a woman's need is for her husband or boyfriend to be affectionate. While on the surface these needs may seem trivial, they are real and can serve as a guide or map to a great relationship.

Other authors on relationships mirror this sentiment. Author John Gray in his work *Mars and Venus Together Forever* states that, more and more, women are living a male role because they are working and competing with men and contributing more to the family finances. However, he states, they still have female needs. While the very real needs of men and women exist, confusion about gender roles creates more friction in relationships. Because of this, it is imperative that couples discuss personal needs in their relationships and accept their partner's needs without judgment. Admitting you have needs is not a weakness; it's a strength. And serving your beloved's needs is love.

7. Understand That Laughter Is the Best Medicine in Good Times and in Bad

Maintaining a great sense of humor can be coupled with not taking yourself so seriously. In the end, most issues are non-issues. When you stop to look at the bigger picture, or step out of the muck you're in, things often look lighter and sometimes even humorous. Saying something witty can break a pattern or jolt someone out of a bad mood. Laughter and lightheartedness are aspects of love.

8. Live by This Principle: No Shame, No Blame, and No Guilt

This goes back to what I've emphasized over and over in this work: *Take responsibility for your actions and reactions.* I once heard the observation that, when you point your finger at someone, four fingers are pointing back at you.

Shame, blame, and guilt are relationship killers. Too many of us carry around our bag of grievances. And when something happens that we don't like, we take out our bag of grievances and begin unloading them onto our loved one.

9. Allow Room for Each Other to Grow

Have you ever heard a married person complain, "But she [or he] is not the person I married." Of course, the person you married, or met, is not the same person. As humans, we are not static. We are ever growing, changing, and developing. It's possible that the person you married did not reveal his or her true self before the marriage. It's also possible that the person you married chose a path that led to self-destructive behaviors. And perhaps he or she is growing but not always according to your expectations. Growth is necessary personally and in relationship. When two people come together as individuals, they meet each other on their individual paths. Even though we come together in relationship to share the journey, we still have to carry out our purpose in life as individuals. Too often, we try to force our loved one onto our path or vice versa. When you allow your beloved to explore his or her own path and you offer support along the way, you are expressing one of the greatest gifts of love.

10. Develop Authentic Expression with One Another

People in healthy relationships feel they can safely express themselves to their loved ones without the threat of putting an end to the relationship or getting hurt. This precious safety net should not be taken lightly. In other words, your loved one feels comfortable opening up to you and expressing feelings, hopes, dreams, and fears. Take this authentic expression as a fragile gift. Too often, people who feel hurt take this information and use it to hurt the other. Or sometimes one member of a couple uses it against the other as a jab, as something to make fun of. Vulnerability is a must in authentic, healthy relationships. But with vulnerability comes great responsibility not to hurt your partner while trying to meet your own needs.

If you are having trouble with authentic expression, or your partner has difficulty opening up, you can try using a few tools, such as the following, to create a safe space for open expression.

PLAN A TIME WHEN ONE PERSON IS GIVING AND THE OTHER IS RECEIVING

This could be a time when you share something you've been meaning to tell your beloved but have been afraid to share. It could be a time when one person gives a massage and the other receives without having to reciprocate. Or it could be a date or other outing fully planned by the giver.

In the case of verbal expression, make sure the giver is sharing without interruption and the receiver is openly receiving the information without giving advice, making faces or commentary, or judging the giver. If it's intimate touch, the receiver shows gratitude toward the partner who's giving, but doesn't feel compelled to return the favor. If the giver has planned something, the receiver appreciates and accepts the gift of what the giver has offered, again with gratitude and without judgment.

IN VERBAL EXPRESSION, REFLECT BACK WHAT YOU HEARD

Usually when receiving information, we are so busy reacting, planning a response, or inferring what has been said that we miss what the other person is actually saying to us. By telling the person what you heard, you clarify any misconceptions or misunderstandings. Many people have difficulty opening up because they are afraid of being misunderstood. When your partner is done talking, you can start your response by saying, "So what you are telling me is…" or "What I heard you say is…"

CREATE A RULE THAT NO INTERRUPTING IS ALLOWED WHILE EITHER IS TALKING

I understand that this one seems obvious, but you'd be amazed at how much you probably interrupt when your partner is speaking. A nice tool you can use to remind yourself not to interrupt is an object the speaker can hold while speaking. Whoever is holding the object may speak, while the other person is required to listen.

Remember one last thing about authentic expression: Expressing yourself honestly and openly to your partner does not mean you are free to hurt. Go back to the lesson taught by Dr. Simon, which I discuss in the section "Cultivating the Act of Witnessing Awareness." There are three gateways between a thought and speaking. In order to speak, you must pass through all three. Ask, "Is what I am about to say true?" If so, proceed to the second gateway. Next ask, "Is what I am about to say necessary?" If so, proceed to the third gateway, and ask yourself, "Is what I am about to say kind?" Once you've passed through all three, you may speak.

11. Do Not Take Each Other for Granted

Appreciate everything you share with your beloved. Maintain a sense of awe and avoid complacency. Say "thank you" often.

Practice gratitude for all the little things in your relationship, and watch it grow.

12. Give without Needing to Receive

Keeping track of who did what is a relationship killer. There will be times in a relationship when you give more than you receive and vice versa. And when you do give, give with love, not out of obligation. If you give out of pure obligation, you taint the giving. Sometimes there are things you do for your beloved that she could, in fact, do for herself. When you find yourself resenting giving in this way, have a conversation and ask your partner if she could pick up the slack in that particular thing. Chances are your partner did not realize it created a burden for you and, when asked nicely, is more than happy to take over the task. Inversely, if there is something you need that you're not receiving, ask for it. Most people are not mind readers. In the following exercise, you can explore ways to communicate your needs effectively and compassionately.

The best way to expand a relationship is to give together: find time to volunteer and help others as a couple. We often get so wrapped up in our own needs and desires that we forget others around us may have even greater or more immediate needs. The bond created in your relationship by giving to others will generate even more gratitude and appreciation in you for what you already have. You realize that this life is not all about you but about serving.

Exercise: Taking Inventory of Your Relationship Using the Twelve Traits

If you are currently in a relationship, go back and look at the Twelve Traits of Healthy Relationships and see where you are. How does your relationship measure up? In what areas do you see room for improvement? Use the following questions to rate your relationship according to each item in that list, and then rate yourself. If your partner is open to doing the exercise with you, then have him or her do the same thing.

1. Does unconditional love exist in the relationship? Do you strive to love unconditionally? What could you do to expand your unconditional love for your partner?

2. Do you find there is mutual acceptance in your relationship? Do you find that you accept your partner as a person no matter what? If not, how can you be more accepting? To accept your loved one, what steps will you have to take?

3. Do you sweat the small stuff? Do you and your partner argue about things such as chores, money, dirty socks, or who takes out the trash? Do you find yourself nitpicking about characteristics or habits of your partner that could be overlooked because they are not that important? If so, how can you turn this around?

4. Is there daily loving touch in your relationship? Do you hug, kiss, and make love and/or stroke each other daily? Is there passion in your touch? Do you love touching your partner? Does he or she perceive you that way? If there is a lack of touch, what are you willing to do to increase touch in your relationship?

5. Do you consistently create great memories together as a couple? Do you gush about fond memories

and plan on creating future memories? Do you focus on the positive or the negative in your relationship? If your focus is more on the negative, how can you emphasize the positive? Where your attention goes, energy flows, so make a commitment to focus on the positive memories in your relationship.

6. Are you aware of each other's needs? Would you be able to list your partner's top five needs that you can fulfill for him or her? If you haven't a clue or can't come up with five, plan on having a conversation with your loved one and asking him or her which needs are in the top five.

7. Do you and your partner laugh together daily? Do you try to lighten the mood by smiling, cracking a joke, or telling a funny story when things get heavy? Do you laugh at yourself in front of your partner regularly? If not, how can you lighten the mood?

8. As a couple, do you make it a practice to assign blame when something goes wrong? Do you remind your partner of his or her shortcomings or past mistakes? Do you consistently point out when your partner is doing something you don't agree with? If so, work on surprising your partner by mentioning what he or she is doing right. Realize that blame need not be assessed in every situation, fix the problem, and move on. Learn to apologize when you do or say something wrong or that hurts the other. Create a plan to let go of blame, shame, and guilt.

9. As a couple, do you allow and encourage each other to grow and have personal-growth time? As a person, do you take time for yourself each day and commit to learning something new on a regular basis? Do you allow your partner to do the same? Write down some ways in which you can support your partner in his or her personal growth.

10. As a couple do you express yourselves authentically to one another, or do you maintain barriers that prevent you from being open, honest, frank, and heartfelt? Do you, as a lover, express yourself to your partner, or do you hold back or sugarcoat things? Do you keep a part of yourself guarded out of fear? Are you afraid to be honest? What steps can you take to open yourself up to your partner authentically?

11. As a couple do you both appreciate each other and all that you do for one another? Do you appreciate that your loved one is in your life? Do you tell him or her on a regular basis? Do you feel gratitude in your heart and thank your creator for the gift of having your loved one in your life? What could you say to your partner to show that you don't take him or her for granted?

12. As a couple do you give to one another without keeping track of who does what? Do you give regularly to your loved one, or are you the one who consistently asks for something? Are you open to receiving? What specifically can you do to give to your partner love, without expecting anything in return?

Communicating Compassionately

A healthy relationship doesn't simply fall into place with ease. It requires work and great communication skills. Communicating is more than expressing yourself and actively listening. It's about expressing yourself effectively and saying what it is that you really need.

When we communicate, we often are trying to fulfill one of our own needs. What we must keep in mind is that the other person too is attempting to have his or her needs met. Can you imagine why people typically have problems with communicating effectively?

Compassionate communication is about being mindful of the other person and his or her needs while effectively communicating yours. There are certain rules you can follow to ease communication and make it successful for you and your partner.

Find a Time to Communicate
When There Are Few or No Distractions

Often we bombard our loved one with conversation when the time isn't right. The TV may be going, kids may be running around, or our partner may be busy with another task. Experience will tell you that distractions plus communication never equals a great result. Either wait until the distraction is no longer an issue or, if it can't wait, look at the person directly and ask, "Can we move to another room for five minutes and have a quick conversation?" If the conversation is about a topic that won't be resolved quickly, ask, "When do you have some time to talk?" You may also offer two options: "Is today after work okay?" or "Tomorrow morning over coffee?"

Respect Your Partner's Style of Communication

The love of my life prefers to do a walk and talk, while I prefer to sit quietly and look at him while talking. This can create a bit of friction when the tension is high. What we are learning to do is to do a little of both. Each person is different in giving and receiving information. Ask your partner if they prefer talking in a quiet environment or a noisy one, if they can talk about a topic in short bits or prefer to have one long conversation and move on. Also, it's important to know your own personal style. Since I'm a writer by nature, I like to write a letter to sort out my thoughts. However, what I learned in the past is that the men in my life didn't necessarily like getting letters, because they're mostly one-sided. Now I write out my thoughts and keep that letter with me during the conversation, and either read it to my partner or highlight key points from it.

Avoid Communicating Important Topics Electronically

This is something new. We live on our devices today, and it's too easy to quickly communicate a thought electronically via text message, voicemail, email, or another form of electric communication. Unfortunately, in our haste we often forget to filter what we say. When your emotions are running high, refrain from sending an emotional message to your loved one.

Understand That Men and Women Communicate and Process Information Differently

When I was teaching middle and high school, we were told to ask a question and wait about thirty seconds before calling on a child. The reason was that boys process questions differently than girls and they need a slightly longer processing time. As a woman, I'm a quick thinker. I ask questions quickly and I want quick answers. Many women I know operate similarly. Men often need a longer reflection time and may need questions asked in a different way. Another difference between men and women is that men are problem solvers. If you present a situation to a man, he will try to find a solution. In communicating compassionately with a man, tell him before you begin, "I need to vent right now. You don't need to solve this. I just need you to listen. Could you do that for me?" That statement allows the man in your life to sit back and listen without the burden of finding a solution. In the event that you need his feedback or advice, after speaking you could say, "I've given you a lot of information; do you need some time to think this over?" If he says yes, give him that time.

Men need to understand that women process information as they speak and often work on solving problems while speaking. So if your lovely woman partner talks a lot and it's not making sense to you, sit back and nod occasionally, or touch her lovingly with a rub on the back or a hand on the knee. Chances are she'll stop talking when she feels better or feels that she's coming to a solution on her own.

There is a four-step process in compassionate communication outlined by Dr. Marshall Rosenberg in his work *Nonviolent Communication: A Language of Life.*[2] This process is relatively simple in concept but a little trickier to put into practice. The process starts with observing what happened and communicating that observation. Observation is like a news reporter describing a scene without emotion, judgments, or inferences. The second step is to identify your feelings — are you feeling angry, happy, sad, frustrated, elated, or stressed?

Then communicate the feeling to your partner. The third step is to identify the need that is not being met: do you need peace, security, love, affection, or appreciation? And the fourth step is to request what you want from the other person. By asking for what we need, we are more likely to receive it. I highly recommend this work because it promotes effective communication.

As we work on our own style of communicating and learn new methods that help us respect the other person, it can seem like we're playing a game, being manipulative, or staging our conversations. In reality, most of us have not learned to communicate our needs because we have not had proper role models. Many of us have been taught not to ask for what we need because it's selfish. And in turn, we've learned to scold others who communicate their needs. So yes, in the beginning it seems staged or awkward. But with practice it becomes less uncomfortable and more fulfilling. The game playing becomes nullified because you are no longer making others guess what you need. As my guru, Dr. Simon, used to say, "Babies cry, and everyone runs around trying to figure out what they need. You now have skills to communicate. So if you cry, fuss, and make others guess at what you want, it doesn't work because you're not that cute anymore."

Minding the Doshas in Relationships

Now that we've ironed out the fact that men and women are different and discussed how to have a healthy relationship, let's take a look at how the doshas can affect our relationships. By understanding that Vata, Pitta, and Kapha types act and react differently, you can find certain propensities in their behavior and learn to work with them.

Vata Types

Vata types are always on the move. They fidget when they sit. They pace when they talk. They are often doing more than one thing at the same time and have a difficult time finishing tasks. Your Vata lover is prone to worry and nervousness and sensitive to mood changes. He may seem hot and cold when it comes to affection. Sometimes the Vata type likes to sit and snuggle, and the next moment he wants to get up and clean the kitchen. Remember the buzzwords for Vata are *change* and *movement*. This can sometimes drive a Pitta or Kapha lover crazy because it seems that there is no consistency. Vata types respond best to touch and sound. Tell your Vata lover that you love her. Touch your Vata lover in the morning and when you come home from work. If you are in a relationship with a Vata type, never blow up at him and leave him thinking about it for the rest of the day. Reassure him that everything will be okay, and then leave. Your Vata's nervous nature will leave the wheels turning, and you will find a crazy person in the evening if you don't reassure him that he need not worry. You can help your Vata lover who is out of balance by cooking her a warm and nourishing meal, drawing a warm bath for her, getting her on a routine, or giving her a shoulder rub before bed. You will always smile because of her enthusiasm, though, and her love for excitement.

Pitta Types

Pitta lovers are intense. They are intense conversationalists and love intensely. Pittas are very attractive for their penetrating gaze and beautiful glowing eyes. They are routine- and goal-oriented. Pitta types can be workaholics, which can make a Vata or Kapha type feel unloved in comparison. Pittas respond best

to the sense of sight: they like their partners to appear beautiful and have impeccable looks. This doesn't necessarily make
them shallow — by nature, they are visual. Dressing nicely,
wearing fine jewelry, or making sure you keep fit for your Pitta
lover will make him happy. A word of caution to those in love
with a Pitta type: Pittas can have a temper. You may notice that
your Pitta lover can be judgmental, critical, or prone to anger.
You may also notice he calms down quickly after spouting off.
If you argue with a Pitta type, you will only add fuel to the fire.
Learn to stay silent or gently remind him at another time that
his words were hurtful, and he'll likely apologize and the warm
fire within him will make you fall for him all over again. In the
bedroom, Pitta types make love passionately and most have a
high sex drive. To help rebalance your Pitta lover, make her a
meal with some cooling foods, such as cucumber, melon, mint,
mango, fennel, or watermelon. Take her to a body of water for
a walk. Dim the lights and listen to some soothing music. Offer
to do a fun activity, which will take her out of her routine.
Make her laugh.

Kapha Types

Kapha lovers are faithful, trustworthy, stable, and nurturing,
and they have great stamina. They adore routine, traditions,
and are great at creating a beautiful home environment. Kapha
types tend to be homebodies and would much rather sit home
by the fire with a good book than be out and about. A Kapha
lover has fantastic stamina in the bedroom and can make love
for the duration. She responds best to the senses of smell and
taste. If you want to please your Kapha lover, buy her a nice
perfume or take her to a five-star restaurant. While your Kapha
lover will not fuss too much, you need to keep in mind that he
takes everything in without complaining but will eventually

withdraw from you when it's too much to handle. Encourage your Kapha lover to consistently share his feelings with you. If you find your Kapha lover getting complacent or too lazy, offer to walk with her. Take her out dancing or to the gym with you. To help your Kapha partner stay in balance, keep sweets out of the house if she complains about weight gain. Eat salads and cook healthy foods with her. You may notice your Kapha lover likes to keep things and that clutter accumulates; tell him you love him and that your relationship is more important to you than any object in the house. An out-of-balance Kapha will need assurance that you won't leave. Give him that and his easygoing nature will surface once again.

Creating the Relationships You Desire

Part of healing is keeping relationships that are nourishing you and letting go of ones that are no longer nourishing. Obviously, there are certain relationships we don't choose consciously, such as those with our children and other immediate family members, but others we can choose.

Regardless of your situation, you can choose to minimize contact with people who bring negative energy to your life. Remember that you also have a conscious choice to allow others to hurt you or not. While physical hurt is never acceptable, psychological or emotional hurt, depending on the situation, can be rectified through compassionate communication or perception. By communicating compassionately, you let others know how you're feeling without attacking them verbally or putting them on the defensive. If a relationship with someone who radiates negativity cannot be avoided, you can choose to perceive that person differently. This will allow you to swallow that bitter pill, so to speak.

What I do when someone is being unkind, judgmental, or harsh is create a story in my head explaining why. For example, I might imagine that the person's spouse just left him, or maybe his mom has been diagnosed with cancer or he himself is dealing with an illness. When I look at the behavior from a different perspective, it helps soften the blow. In reality, we really don't know what another person is dealing with in life. Often when we allow ourselves to get hurt in a relationship, we're thinking it's all about us. We think, "Oh, she did this to me," or "He is out to hurt me." In fact, it's usually about them. Have you ever inadvertently hurt someone and, when you were told this, you had no idea that you had done so? You thought you were just going about your business. Instead, you may have said something wrong or in a way that differed from your usual approach, and the other person took it poorly. So when we shift our perception and recognize that the problem is probably not about us, this takes the burden off our shoulders and helps to turn a tense relationship into a more nourishing one.

Another way to shift perception is by asking questions. Have you ever assumed someone was doing something and then found that you were dead wrong? Instead of saying, "Oh, I know you were out drinking with your buddies last night!" ask, "So what did you end up doing last night?" without an accusative tone, of course. If a friend forgot to call and you assume she doesn't like you anymore, say, "Hey, it looks like you've been busy lately. Did you forget to call?" Other questions you can ask to clarify the speaker's intention might be: "What did you mean by that?" "Did I hear you say...?" "In other words, are you saying...?" Allow the person to clarify, and believe her. You may not believe it now, but by simply shifting from assumptions to questions you can nourish relationships and create better ones.

If you are searching for a partner in life, you can create the relationship you desire and attract the ideal mate into your life. The process is actually easier than we usually assume. I'm sure you've had the experience of searching for a job or a house. Before beginning you usually have an idea of what job you want or living space you'd like. So you create a list, mentally or physically, of things you'd like to have. Then you collect data and determine which companies to send résumés to or which houses to visit. Unless you're in a desperate situation, you typically sort through the choices and make an educated choice based on a lot of criteria. Some of us act on impulse (Vata types are known for this), but most realize that a job choice or house is a big decision. Finding a mate should feel no different. We tend to make it seem different, but in rationally choosing you can attract the right person for you and create a healthy relationship.

Steps to Attract the Right Mate

Tons of books have been written on the subjects of attracting a partner and maintaining an intimate relationship, and this book is certainly not one of them. However, based on my own reading and experience, coupled with a consciousness-based approach, I can offer steps in beginning the process.

1. **WRITE DOWN EVERYTHING YOU WISH TO HAVE IN A MATE.** This process is similar to the one you used to compile your list of intentions and desires. State the sentences in the present tense and in the positive. "The man [or woman] of my dreams is…" Don't hold back. Take an unlimited time to write as much as you can, describing your potential mate.

2. **WRITE DOWN EVERYTHING YOU ABSOLUTELY DON'T WANT IN A MATE.** For example: "He cannot smoke." "She cannot be a couch potato."

3. **Visualize your mate-to-be.** Even if you're not the creative type, you no doubt have read books and seen movies. Imagine you are with your mate. What does she look like, smell like, feel like? What does he wear? What is her occupation? What do you two do on the weekends? In the evenings? On holidays? How do you speak to one another? Visualize absolutely everything and write it down. I did this before meeting my love, and after meeting and dating him for a few months, I went back and read my visualization. It was amazingly close to who my love turned out to be as a person and how we are in our relationship.

4. **Become the kind of person you wish to attract into your life.** Suppose you place honesty at the top of your list of must-have qualities. If your future partner must be honest, then you must hold yourself to the same standard. To paraphrase a quote I once read: "You don't attract what you want; you attract what you are."

5. **Start looking for your mate.** Online dating is very common today, but get out there too. When I was looking for my love, I started going out and salsa dancing. I also went to singles meet-up groups. As hard as it was for me, with three children and a business, I made sure I got out there. It gave a message to the universe: "Hey, I'm available here." Go back to the analogy of searching for a job or a house. When looking for work, I bet you search a lot of different avenues, not just one. You might call past managers; ask friends, neighbors, and past colleagues; post your résumé online; and so on. If you stick to one outlet in a job search, it might take a lot longer. Searching for a mate is no different.

6. **DON'T COMPROMISE YOUR DESIRES LIST AND SETTLE FOR LESS.** Granted, no one is perfect, but just because someone is interested in you doesn't mean you must cave in for fear that no one else is out there. Your mate's characteristics should match a majority of those on your desires list and should not be one that you specifically don't want.

7. **MEDITATE DAILY AND SURRENDER TO THE UNIVERSE.** Stay steadfast in the belief that your ideal mate is out there. You have to trust and believe, without a shadow of a doubt, that he or she is coming into your life. I constantly repeat to my single friends who feel desperate: "Are you kidding me? With 7.5 billion people out there, you're telling me it's hopeless? Your love is out there. He's available and searching for you too. You just have to believe it." Surrender. Ask God, in the form in which you conceive of him or her, to send you your ideal mate. Then watch for clues and follow your intuition.

✔ Checklist for Health

Healing Your Relationships

❑ Explore your relationship with yourself. Are you the person you'll want to be once you're in a relationship with another person? Do you feel you are whole?

❑ Read over the Twelve Traits of Healthy Relationships.

❑ Work on your inventory for the "Twelve Traits of Healthy Relationships," and discover how your relationship measures up.

❑ Do you communicate compassionately? Do you possess a good vocabulary for expressing your feelings?

❑ If you are in a relationship, which dosha is your loved one? How can you cater to his or her dominant dosha within the relationship?

❑ If you are seeking a relationship, write down all the traits you desire in a mate. Do you emulate the qualities of the person you wish to attract? Remember, like attracts like.

CHAPTER EIGHT

OCCUPATIONAL HEALTH

*Choose a job you love and you will never have to work
a day in your life.*

— CONFUCIUS

We spend more time at our job than at any other activity except, perhaps, for sleep. According to a 1999 government study, Americans spend, on average, forty-seven hours a week at work; and 20 percent of all Americans spend an average of forty-nine hours a week working.[1]

And in a 2012 study by the University College London, occupational stress was found to increase the risk of heart attack and accelerate the aging process.[2] Another 2012 study shows that job-related stress increases the risk of diabetes in women.[3]

It is imperative that we heal this aspect of ourselves if we are to experience a balanced life. If you are in a job or vocation you love, then great. You may not need the information in this chapter. But if you are dissatisfied with your job or occupation, then your health, and perhaps your life, depends on changing your situation or your beliefs about your situation. Your job or occupation may be tied to dharma, but it doesn't have to be. If you haven't yet worked through the chapter on dharma, I suggest you go back and address that chapter before continuing with this one.

The Daily Grind

Many of us do our job because we have to. We have to pay the bills, buy clothes and food, and take care of incidentals. Most who are dissatisfied with their jobs find that they are bound by what I call golden handcuffs. They tell themselves, *You have a job, so you should feel grateful, with unemployment the way it is and all. At least you have something to pay the bills.* Those are the golden handcuffs. And those are the people who suffer the most. They usually experience poor physical health as well as psychological disorders such as anxiety or depression. We typically do our jobs because we have to. The French have a colloquial phrase that describes the typical Parisian lifestyle: *Metro, boulot, dodo,* which translates to: "Metro, work, sleep." If you find yourself in this position, either stuck for monetary reasons or simply stuck in a rut, it may be time to make a shift.

Doing What You Love and Loving What You Do

When it comes to your occupation, you have two choices: love the current job situation or learn to love it; or find a new occupation you do love.

Loving what you do may entail a shift in perspective. You could be a person who picks up the trash and finds reasons to love your job. Let's suppose this is the case; then this may be your rationale: "The early morning hours are great. I get to see the sunrise. I get to have the afternoons off to be with the kids. I get to clean up the streets and make them look good." It doesn't matter what job you have; if you believe you are making a difference, you are. For a few years, I went to a certain grocery store near my home and often was served by a checkout lady who was an absolute gem. Every time I saw her, she was wearing a grin from ear to ear. She looked me in the eyes while speaking, and her own eyes glowed. It was so surprising to me because, well, she was a grocery store checkout lady. What did she have to be so happy about? But it was clear to me and everyone who went through her line that she loved her work. And that made me seek her checkout line every single time I went to that store. She made my day just by being cheerful.

If you are unhappy with your place of employment or vocation, can you find ways to love it? Take a good look at your current situation and decide whether, by shifting your perspective, you can love your work.

Let's suppose the answer is no, that you cannot figure out a way to love what you're doing. In that case, it's time for change.

Discovering the Higher Purpose of Having a Career

All the world's a stage,
and all the men and women merely players.

— WILLIAM SHAKESPEARE

Usually people are dissatisfied by their work when they feel they aren't making a difference, either in their workplace or in the lives of others who are affected by the work. We've determined that you spend a great portion of your life in your career; so how do you make it meaningful?

You get to create your life and your career. There are infinite possibilities if you know what you desire. Just as the Shakespeare quote tells us, you and I are playing roles in life; and in your career you get to determine which role to strive for. Write your own script. Any limitations are simply in your mind, in the mental tapes you play back to yourself.

Before starting the Ayurvedic Path Yoga and Wellness Studio, I had had no previous business experience. I knew nothing of marketing, running a business, sales, and accounting, and I hadn't yet been trained in yoga, meditation, and Ayurveda. When I announced to my then husband that I was going to start a business, he was skeptical. He assured me I was reaching so far out of my league that I would certainly fail. And he scoffed when I told him I planned to spend around twenty thousand dollars getting the training I needed in order to even think about starting a business. He lent me the money, believing the whole time I was nothing but a dreamer. His reaction was normal. If you truly look at this, you'll see that all the odds were against me. One thing going for me was that I believed I could do it. I had changed my mental state from doubt to believing that I could start this business, and that I had to. I am proud to say that, six years into it, my business is successful. The road hasn't been easy, and I've made mistakes along the way. But I can say with absolute certainty that I love my work and go to my studio every day with a smile on my face.

In my case my work is my dharma, or purpose in life. But does this mean that your job, the one paying most of the bills, must be your dharma? Not necessarily. For now, your passion or talent may not be sufficient to allow you to pay the bills with your dream job. And that's fine. You can construct your life in a way where you have your day job but you also have your dharma, which you pursue by moonlighting. Let me illustrate with some examples.

One of my aunts spent almost thirty years of her life as a successful manager of a hardware store. Her husband spent about the same amount of time as an engineer for an automobile company. Both of them retired after accumulating enough in their pensions to make ends meet. In retirement they took up a hobby, woodcrafting. They make the most beautiful objects out of wood. After crafting many objects, they go to craft shows and sell their products. They don't make and sell these crafts because they have to; they do it because they love creating them.

Another story is about my sister's friend. By day, he is a curator at a museum. By night he makes cuffs, which are a type of bracelet made of old leather belts and metal studs. He started out making them for friends, and when he realized that so many people wanted them, he decided to sell them for a profit. Since he gets his materials at thrift stores and hardware stores, he makes each cuff for only pennies. He gets a return that is twenty times his monetary investment. He sells his cuffs on weekends at art shows and makes more money that way than he makes in his career.

These two examples illustrate people with artistic abilities, but your talents may lie in something else. I know people who adore gardening, cooking, or serving the poor. If you know what you love to do, but can't figure out a way to make a career out of it, keep your day job. But then it's even more important that you choose a satisfying job, so you'll have the energy to practice your talent or passion once you finish work.

Finding Dharma in a Career
That Is Not Exactly Your Dharma

Dharma is the way we use our God-given talents to serve others. My dharma is to teach others to live healthfully and to live their lives to their fullest potential. If I didn't have my current career, could I still do this? The answer is: "Yes, absolutely!" In fact, I've done it all my life without realizing it. Once you've figured out your dharma by working through the exercises in the chapter on dharma, or if you already know it, you can apply it to any life situation. My daughter is an excellent illustrator and artist. She has created posters for clubs at school, made costumes from scratch for animé conventions, and illustrated cards for family members' birthdays and holidays. Without actually having made art into her career (she decided to pursue another career path), she is using her God-given talents to make everyone around her happy with the beauty of her creations.

Let's suppose your passion lies in taking care of pets. Couldn't you create a pet-sitting service for your coworkers who go out of town for a weekend or longer vacation? You can spread the news that you're willing to take care of pets, for a fee, at your home. In the end, you will be fulfilling your need to express your dharma but also filling the needs of others who want to take a break without worrying about Fido. Can you imagine the warm, fuzzy feelings you'll create even at the workplace?

The possibilities are endless.

Imagine your dharma is cooking. At your day job you could start a fund among coworkers, asking them to put twenty dollars each in the pot for colleagues who are experiencing illness, or who just had a baby or death in the family, and who may not have the energy to cook for themselves. You gather the funds and cook a couple of delicious meals for those coworkers in need and fashion a card to be signed by everyone who donated. You get to express your talent, you help those in need, and you create a sense of community in the workplace.

I know a woman whose dharma is teaching yoga. She went to her company's human resources office and offered to teach a free, lunchtime yoga class once a week.

Now that your creative juices are no doubt flowing, let's explore how your Ayurvedic mind-body type figures into occupational health.

Honoring Your True Nature:
Ideal Work for Vata, Pitta, Kapha

Your prakruti, or your true nature, will determine to some degree what type of work will keep you in balance.

Vata Types

Since Vata types are governed by the air and space elements, they tend to enter creative or communications fields. Vatas are often artists, writers, actors, or otherwise in the creative field. They also gravitate toward careers in which they deal with people, such as marketing and sales or human resources. Since routine keeps a Vata type in balance, they need to be careful about jobs with erratic schedules, night shifts, and jobs that require frequent travel. While Vatas thrive in new and exciting environments, too much change will pull a Vata out of balance. Working in a somewhat structured environment — which can be arranged even in a creative field — will keep a Vata type balanced.

ADVICE TO A VATA TYPE: Stay grounded and focused. Don't leave a job simply for the change. If you experience boredom daily, see if you can move to a different job at your company or place of work. Changing jobs frequently will only imbalance your life, however. While you may crave change, it is sometimes your worst enemy. When you get absorbed in a project, set an alarm on your phone or computer to remind yourself to take a break and eat something. Going for a walk midday will help make use of some of the restless Vata energy and help you remain focused for the rest of your day.

Pitta Types

Composed of fire and water, Pitta types are intense and goal oriented. They adore education, learning facts, and sharing their knowledge with the world. Pittas are often seen in leadership positions. They are good as educators, politicians, lawyers, and doctors. Balanced Pitta types make strong leaders, since they are organized, precise, and orderly. They are warm and eloquent speakers. Pittas are extremely bright but can also become controlling and dominating. They need to balance their leadership skills with courses or workshops in effective management, which will teach them compassion for others. Otherwise they can become overbearing in the workplace. Pitta types need to be careful when they enter a highly competitive work environment. Because of their competitive nature, they can wind up working too many hours, stressing too much over work, and developing excess stomach acid, ulcers, or heart disease. A wise and balanced Pitta will learn to say no from time to time in order to create room, in her busy work schedule, for exercise, family, and leisure.

ADVICE TO A PITTA TYPE: Realize that, in the workplace, not many people will be perfectionists like you. That doesn't mean they don't have a good work ethic; it simply means their standards are not the same as yours. Instead of criticizing others for not living up to your expectations, offer one or two pieces of constructive criticism with a concrete request related to each item. Also, realize that work will not bring you the greatest amount of happiness, because you will always seek more. Make sure you maintain a healthy life outside of work. Nourish friendships and family life. Take time to immerse yourself in nature. Make time for prayer and spiritual practice, which will help you relinquish some of your need for control.

Kapha Types

Methodical, meticulous, and *stable* are all words describing Kapha. Kapha types, who are composed of water and earth, are reliable in any organization. Since they don't enjoy change, finding a career in which they are happy is essential. A Kapha will stay in a job even if she doesn't enjoy it, because stability is more important than happiness. A Kapha is often a great complement to a Pitta boss, because the Kapha employee is kind, loving, and forgiving. Generally, he's not going to let the temper of a Pitta get to him. Kaphas enjoy work that is not too rushed, since their nature is to do things slowly and thoroughly. They have great stamina and can work long hours without getting too tired.

ADVICE TO A KAPHA TYPE: At the workplace, learn to say no from time to time. Your sweet nature predisposes you to take on too much simply because others rely on you. Your coworkers know you're dependent and trustworthy. They also know you're nice and kind. Without meaning to, they may take advantage of that niceness. Even though you know you can handle it because of your fantastic stamina, you will accumulate resentment and feel the weight of too much work on your shoulders. The weight will cause you to eat too much or become depressed. By saying no when you are feeling overwhelmed, you will keep yourself in balance. Another way to stay healthy is to create a walking club at work and walk with coworkers on your lunch breaks. When you stimulate your Kapha body and get things moving, you will feel stronger and have greater ability to assert yourself.

Exercise: Creating a Plan for Transforming Your Current Job or Finding Your Ideal Job

Answer the following questions and begin thinking about how you will transform your occupational health.

1. Am I satisfied with my current job? Why? Why not?

2. What is my dharma, or purpose in life?

3. Is my current work situation fulfilling my dharma? If not, can I find a way to fulfill my dharma in my current job? Why? Why not?

4. What things must I have in my ideal job? Think about environment, job position, workload, hours, pay, benefits, company vision, management, vacation time, distance from home, and so on.

5. How can I create my ideal job? And how can I integrate my dharma into my job?

Here is a list of my intentions for my career, occupation, or vocation:

✔ Checklist for Health

A Healthy Occupation

❏ Do you love what you do? Can you?

❏ What is the higher purpose of a career for you?

❏ How can you find dharma in a career that is not exactly your dharma?

❏ Explore how your career can accommodate your Ayurvedic mind-body type.

❏ Complete the exercise Creating a Plan for Transforming Your Current Job or Finding Your Ideal Job.

CHAPTER NINE

FINANCIAL HEALTH

Money isn't everything....
But it ranks right up there with oxygen.

— RITA DAVENPORT

Finances! This is one of the most emotionally charged topics ever. And it's a topic necessary for all of us to address, regardless of our situation. For centuries it was taboo to talk of finances and impolite to ask others about their salaries. Money was something talked about behind closed doors or maybe not even discussed at all. In America, until the 1950s, husbands took care of the household finances, giving their wives an allowance to use for the week. Generous husbands gave their wives money for the groceries and the children's expenses, and maybe a few dollars on the side so the women could get their hair done. But women who didn't work did not have a safety net in case their husbands died or left them. With women in the workplace, things have changed, but our knowledge of finances and money hasn't.

According to an analysis of Federal Reserve statistics and other government data, as of 2014 the average household owes $7,274 on their credit cards.[1] But if we take into account only the indebted households, those numbers change to an average of $15,593 in household credit card debt, $153,184 in mortgage debt, and $32,511 on student loan debt. Twenty-five percent of U.S. households have more credit card debt than emergency savings.[2] The message is clear: when it comes to finances, we have a serious problem.

Your Financial Situation and Your Health

Do not fool yourself into believing your finances do not affect your health. Have you ever in your life worried about money? Have you ever wondered where you would get the money to pay the next bill, cover the rent or mortgage, or fix the broken car? Have you felt the discomfort in talking with your spouse about money, cringing at the thought that it may even start an argument? Even if you're doing fine financially, have you ever gotten upset after lending money to a friend or family member in need, only to have them never pay you back?

Increased stress leads to increases in stress hormones, ulcers, a depressed immune system, and higher blood pressure. Worries about money affect relationships and our emotional well-being.

Money affects us on every level. And our belief about money guides us in ways that we sometimes don't even understand. Our upbringing taught us a fair amount about money even if it wasn't talked about. But most of us haven't been formally taught how to manage it.

According to Ayurveda, money is energy; and part of our duty is to attract it into our life without greed. Artha, or the accumulation of wealth as a householder — and one of the four aims of life — is regarded as a necessity. Money flows in and out of our lives. It's actually an ebb and flow. But with our own will, desires, and anxiety or fear, we can prevent the two-way flow of money, wealth, and abundance in our lives. Therefore, we must stay mindful of our thoughts and actions surrounding money, avoiding either holding on to it too tightly or spending it unwisely.

The doshas rule our natural propensities regarding money and wealth, to some extent. Vata types make money easily but also spend it easily, especially on trivialities, and they often find themselves broke. Pitta types work hard to accumulate money and wealth but also have expensive tastes: they enjoy spending money on luxuries. Kapha types are good at saving and holding on to their money.

Getting Rid of a Poverty Mind-Set

Most of us have been brought up with poverty consciousness, a mind-set that says, "I don't have enough." You've heard people say things like: "Money doesn't grow on trees," "We can't afford it," "I'm living paycheck to paycheck," and "Once I win the lottery, I'll start enjoying life." Do you realize that by thinking you won't have enough, you won't?

I grew up in a household where my mother incessantly told us we were poor. We always heard: "We're poor; we can't afford it." She literally conditioned us to believe it. I hated hearing those words. But internally, I never really believed them. Yes, she was a single mother and had had to wait tables to put herself through college and pay the bills. But here's the startling thing: even when she was a seasoned schoolteacher making seventy thousand dollars a year, she still said she was poor. The mind-set never changed. At nineteen, when I began to travel the world, I saw real poverty. I realized that in the United

States we're not poor. While we may say we're poor, we have a roof over our heads, a television, and a car. According to other countries in the world, we are rich. Perspective is everything.

Poverty mind-set poisons abundance and wealth consciousness. I once saw a special edition of the *Oprah Winfrey Show*, which she had recorded in India. She visited a home in the slums of Mumbai, where she found a family of four — a husband, wife, and two daughters — living in a hundred-square-foot home. Now imagine, the entire home measured ten feet by ten feet. In that home, they prepared meals, ate, played, and slept. The bathroom was outdoors. The husband went to work on a moped and spent much of his earnings to send his daughters to private school. Here's the surprising part: they had few material possessions and necessities, but they were happy. They considered themselves not poor but middle class.

You can have little money but feel rich, and you can have an abundance of money and feel poor. It is all about the way you think.

Exercise: Taking Stock of Your Beliefs about Money

Be honest with yourself as you complete the following prompts. There are no right or wrong answers. Simply be aware of your beliefs. Once you have this awareness, you can choose to keep your beliefs or change them.

1. When I was growing up, I believed the following about money:

2. Phrases my parents or other caretakers repeated to me about money:

3. Now my current financial situation is:

4. Phrases about money that I repeat to myself now:

Honoring Money as Energy: Giving to Receive

As I mentioned, poverty consciousness and wealth consciousness are mind-sets. Even if you're stuck in poverty consciousness, you can train your mind to replace it with abundance consciousness. It's not an easy thing to do, but with consistent training it's possible.

Practicing Gratitude

I've mentioned this already, but it bears repeating: being thankful for what is already in your life is the best way to notice wealth and abundance. Every day, say thank you to your creator, thank your spouse or lover and your children for being in your life. Thank your friends, colleagues, and anyone who touches your life. Notice how much you have in your life already, even if your bank account is empty. Look at your home, your furniture, your car, your clothing, your dishes, your clean drinking water — everything in your life. Then expand this consciousness to encompass the earth. Gaze at the sun, notice the birds, the trees, the flowers, the animals. Appreciate nature's beauty and your ability to appreciate it. Give thanks for your five senses, your limbs, and for your health. You are truly blessed and abundant.

Giving to Others

You may wonder how giving is going to make you rich and abundant. Remember that money is energy, and what you give out comes back to you. Every religion teaches about giving. Everything I've read about creating wealth states the same thing, that you must give a portion of what you have if money is to come to you. Many philosophies believe that you should give 10 percent of your gross earnings, which means before taxes. Financial guru Suze Orman states in her book *The 9 Steps to Financial Freedom* that you should ask your inner voice how much to give. If your inner voice says 5 percent, heed that inner wisdom. If your inner voice tells you to give 10 percent and you give only 5 percent, you will retain your poverty consciousness. Trusting that there is enough will prove to you there is. When you hold back, frightened by the prospect that you will lack sufficient money, you continue to embrace poverty and wear its shackles.

Let me share a story about an experience I had in France. While in college, I was staying with a French family who would be considered middle class by European standards. They lived well but were not rich. While I stayed there, we always ate very well. We would begin the meal with a small appetizer followed by a vegetable, such as grilled asparagus with dressing. Next came the meat dish, which consisted of a piece of meat divided among all those seated at the table, including the guests. Then we always ate a small salad, yogurt or cheese, and a piece of fruit for dessert. Throughout the meal, we had pieces of baguette. What surprised me was that the main dish, the meat or fish, was always cut to accommodate the guests. If another guest showed up, no problem; everyone's share simply got a little smaller. The host wouldn't flinch at all and would simply make do. She would never apologize for not having enough food, but would feel proud to allow into her home, and feed, whoever was there.

When I returned to the United States, I noticed how

differently people would approach the same situation. If a host didn't have a steak for each person, she would either go out and buy more or invite fewer people. In her mind, there wasn't enough. Do you see how the French family exhibited the consciousness of abundance?

My experience taught me to put generosity into practice. I am committed to giving away 10 percent of my income before I spend it on anything else, including bills. Orman suggests writing your check for the charity or person you're giving it to before you receive your pay; that way you're even more committed. When you receive your pay, send your gift right away. But of course, never get into debt in order to give. In other words, don't put your gift on your credit card if you cannot pay off that bill straightaway.

Exercise: A Commitment to Financial Giving

Some religions call financial giving tithing. The idea is to give a portion of your income to a charitable cause. In this exercise, you will decide how much you will give and who you will give it to. And if you're not sure now how much you can afford, commit to giving some amount and then readjust it later.

How much are you committed to giving?

Who will you give to?

Finally, giving is always between you and your creator. Never fret about where the money is going to go or how it will be spent. Do your research and choose wisely, but in the end you are giving to give. Your gift must be unconditional for it to work. You are sending the message to the universe that the money isn't really yours anyway. It's a gift, just like what you are giving away.

Your Plan to Abolish Debt and Create Wealth in Your Life

We have now ascertained that your health is directly linked to your financial state. And debt can weigh you down and keep you in servitude to your creditors. If you have no debt, congratulations! You are doing a great job financially. You can skip over this section, or you can read it to make sure you never let yourself go into debt.

Most of us in the United States have a certain amount of debt, whether it is credit card debt, a car loan, a mortgage, or personal debt. I've read many books on personal finance, and a couple of authors I've found helpful are Ric Edelman and Suze Orman. I recommend reading some of their books if you'd like to do a complete personal-finance overhaul. But for now, here are a few pointers to get you started on abolishing debt.

1. Make a List of All Your Debts and Get Real about the Amounts

No use hiding from yourself. You will have to pay those debts anyway. Keep the debtor, amount due, and minimum payments due on a spreadsheet.

2. Start Paying Off the Small Debts First

When you pay off a small debt, you can compound your payments on larger debts. This is a psychological move I learned from Ric Edelman. It may seem illogical to wipe out the smaller debt first when the higher debts may have higher interest rates. What Edelman explains is that our psyche gets excited about wiping out a debt, and in the long run it will actually become easier to pay off all debts this way. Let me give you an example:

Let's say you owe $252 to a department store, $455 to Visa, and $2,400 on your MasterCard. The minimum payments are as follows: $25, $35, and $75. You know you can add $50 extra to get rid of your debts. You will then pay $75 to the department store, $35 to Visa, and $75 to MasterCard. You will continue to do this until the department store card is paid off. Now, we're assuming that you are not accumulating any more debt on any of these cards in the meanwhile. Once you've eradicated the debt on the department store card, you will take the $75 and apply it each month to the Visa card. Your payments will now be $110 to Visa and $75 to MasterCard. You are still paying $185 total — but do you see that it looks much better to be able to pay more toward the second credit card once the first is paid off? After the Visa card is paid off, apply the whole $185 to MasterCard.

3. Never Stay Indebted to Friends and Family

Your family and your friends are your lifelines. If you borrow money from them, pay them off first. Joe's Plumbing or American Express can wait. They are companies and have no investment in your personal life. Yes, they are charging interest, but relationships are more important than money. Value your relationships and the trust you have developed there. Even if friends or family say to you, "It's no big deal; pay me when you can," believe me, it is a big deal. Your integrity, your trustworthiness, and your self-worth all lie in the fact that you can and will repay your family and friends who had the kindness to lend to you.

4. Pay Yourself First

This concept I learned from motivational speaker and author Anthony Robbins. Set aside amounts each month that you will invest, that you will add to your retirement fund, and that you will add to your emergency savings. Time is money, and the sooner you invest in yourself, the more time your money will have to compound.

5. Do Not Forgo Your Retirement Fund to Save for Your Children's College Tuition

Orman explains that this is the biggest mistake most parents make. If you do not save for your retirement, who will save for you, and who will take care of you financially when you do retire? If there is a choice between saving for your children's college tuition and investing money for retirement, always choose retirement. Your children, after college, will be young enough and have the potential for earning that you will not have. They can take on the burden of student loans if there isn't any other choice. You, on the other hand, will have nothing, and no one to rely on, during your retirement years. If the money isn't here now, it won't be there when you retire.

6. Educate Yourself and Begin Talking about Money

The more you read about personal finance, the less you will fear it. I have a recommended-reading list at the end of this book that will help you get started. The books listed there are my personal favorites, and I'm sure you will find them useful and their principles easy to apply.

Talking about money, as I mentioned, makes most people uncomfortable. If you share expenses with someone, such as a spouse, partner, or family member, start the conversation.

Realize that the more comfortable you become while talking about money, the easier it will become. When you begin the conversation, state the fact that there is nothing innately personal about money. It's an object, a concept, and energy — and that's all. It is not tied to our personalities, so no one should get offended. You and your spouse, partner, or family member may have different beliefs about money, but make a pact stating that the goal is to create healthy spending patterns, not to give or take personal jabs.

If you have children, talk to them often about money. Give them a little money to manage, and explain to them about giving and investment. Children as young as five can understand the concept of money. Be mindful of the conversations about money that you have around your children and the catch-phrases you use. Remember, your children are listening to you and forming their own beliefs about money.

7. Celebrate Money by Designating Fun Money

Often when we feel a sense of lack, we punish ourselves by paying everyone else and maybe investing but not treating ourselves to something nice or fun. You work hard for your money. If you can't enjoy it, then what's it all for? Set aside each month an amount that seems reasonable to you and simply have fun with it. Buy that hundred-dollar pair of shoes you've been wanting. Get a great massage. Take a couple friends out to an upscale restaurant. Stay within your fun-money budget, but enjoy it without guilt.

If we don't do this, we create a rubber-band effect. We hold back and deprive ourselves so much that the rubber band snaps and we find ourselves going wild. We feel so deprived that we go out and charge a thousand dollars on the credit card all at once. Then, after doing that, we feel bad and return to deprivation mode. Can you see the destructive pattern? So make the decision today about the amount you can designate as your fun money. If you're married, and one parent stays at home with the children, that parent gets fun money too. When I was married we called this don't-ask money. Each of us put an equal amount into the household budget, and we could do whatever we wanted with it. The other person could not ask, under any circumstances, what the money was spent on. It could have been a hundred chocolate bars. It didn't matter. We all deserve to create a healthy balance in our finances.

✔ Checklist for Health
Healing Your Finances

❑ Take a look at your finances today. Do you believe your financial state can be affecting your health?

❑ What is your mind-set concerning money? For you, does money have a positive connotation or a negative one?

❑ Practice gratitude daily for all the things you have.

❑ Give something to someone each day. Train your brain to be 100 percent certain that there is more than enough money to go around.

❑ Create a plan to abolish any debt you may have.

❑ Pick out two books on personal finance and begin reading them.

❑ If you share expenses with someone, plan a conversation about healthy spending or budgeting.

❑ Designate an amount for your fun money and stick to it.

CHAPTER TEN

ENVIRONMENTAL HEALTH

The environment is everything that isn't me.

— ALBERT EINSTEIN

According to Ayurveda, the environment is your extended body. Anything outside your physical body is an extension of you. Imagine that! In the West, when we speak about environment we usually refer to it as a movement of some sort. We have to be *environmentally friendly* — that is, reduce our carbon footprint by recycling, driving vehicles with low or zero emissions, and reusing bags and boxes. We ponder things like global warming and the melting polar ice caps. Ayurveda expands this definition to include absolutely everything outside of you. And when you stop to think about it, the Ayurvedic definition creates a greater sense of responsibility and greater awareness of how you choose to create your life.

Our environment includes our homes, cars, rooms, office space, the people we know, the places we visit, and, of course, the entire earth and universe. Some aspects of our environment we can control directly, and others we cannot. In this chapter we will explore ways you can control your various environments in order to make yourself healthier and happier.

Our sensory experience is a great part of our health. When I was on the road to healing, I read a wonderful book by Dr. Andrew Weil titled *8 Weeks to Optimum Health*. In one of the exercises, he recommended buying flowers for yourself. At first this seemed absurd. I believed that flowers were something you gave to others and that others gave to you. But I followed through, and every week for eight weeks, I bought myself a bouquet of flowers. And you wouldn't believe the effect of simply having fresh flowers in my kitchen. I was so happy every time I walked in there. It lifted my mood and made me want to clean my kitchen so that the flowers would look even prettier. Can you believe I cleaned my kitchen for a bouquet of flowers? And that is just one aspect of environment.

Through Dr. Weil's book, I also learned about minimizing unnecessary sensory input, and to this day, fifteen years later, I'm still following that advice. Ayurveda mimics this sentiment. Be careful about what you let into your sensory perception. We are bombarded daily with sights and sounds and don't even realize the implications for our health.

I'm referring to simple things, from watching the news to seeing continual advertising on the computer. At home we may live with the constant drone of the television or radio. And some people go to bed at night with their TV sets on and leave them on all night. We are affected by violence and negative imagery even though we may not consciously perceive them. An absence of silence can make us jittery, nervous, and unfocused. The constant flicker of a TV at night disrupts the release of the hormone melatonin, which requires complete darkness.

Maximizing Healthy Sensory Input

Healing can come when you pay close attention to each of the five senses and consciously choose stimuli that heal. Each of the five senses also corresponds to a dosha.

Taste

Choose fresh, organic, local foods. Surround yourself with fresh bowls of fruit. Make sure each plate of food is colorful and well presented, even if you're feeding only yourself. Take time to taste your food and chew it slowly, and keep quiet while you savor each bite. Ayurveda recommends we get each of the six tastes in our meals, even if we are taking supplemental herbs. A mind-body connection is made when the body perceives taste. When we are aware of taste, we are likely to eat less. When we appreciate taste and select only desirable tastes on a conscious level, we are less apt to choose unhealthy, artificial, or greasy food. Have you ever bitten into a freshly picked apple or apricot? The sensation in the body is much different than if you truly taste something like a fast-food French fry. Try it some time. Close your eyes and taste a fresh, healthy food, and do the same with an unhealthy food. The healthier and more aware you become, the more likely you will reject the unhealthy food. I've done this with my kids. I've trained them to appreciate fine foods. Now that they are teenagers, when they taste an unhealthy food, they know the difference and reject it. Your body is an environment and the sense of taste is important to keeping your body free of toxins.

Smell

The sense of smell is closely linked to the sense of taste. Have you ever eaten something when you had a cold and then discovered you couldn't properly taste it? Usually it's difficult to taste anything when your nose is stuffed up. Keep your environments smelling pleasant for you. We all have neuroassociations with the sense of smell, since it's a strong and primal sense. Find a perfume you enjoy, and others will enjoy on you too. You'll know because people will say to you, "You smell so good!" It makes you feel good and others too. In your bedroom, find a pleasant, sleep-inducing scent. Some people like lavender, jasmine, or chamomile. Home cooking induces a sense of peace and well-being in the home. Allowing soups or stews to simmer in the winter, or having a barbecue in the summer, seems to bring about pleasant memories and create strong neuroassociations with the surrounding environment.

In my own experience, I had a blast from the past when I entered an Indian restaurant about ten years ago. At that time, I had eaten few Indian dishes. But I was with my sister and dad, and we walked into an Indian restaurant to eat. The smells took me back to my aunt's kitchen. I couldn't get enough of the smell. It made me feel happy, comfy, cozy, safe, and secure. Imagine a smell that can do all that! My father is from the Middle East, and what I realized was that the spices in Indian cooking are the same as the spices used in Middle Eastern cooking. To me, the smells of spices meant more than simply good food. They meant the love of family, comfort, and the roots of culture and tradition.

Think about the smells you want in your environment. Perhaps fresh flowers? A favorite bread you like to bake? A dish you're famous for in your family? Remember, you are creating memories for everyone via the smells you choose to have around you. Make sure they're pleasant for your family, other loved ones, and yourself.

While everyone responds well to taste and smell, Kapha types respond most strongly to them, since these senses are dominant in the Kapha mind-body type. If Kapha is your predominant dosha, pay extra attention to these two.

Hearing

Does it amaze you that you can hear a song you haven't heard in twenty years and still sing the lyrics? Or is there a jingle from a commercial in your past that you can still sing to this day, even though it hasn't aired in years? I will bet you answered yes to both questions. Our sense of hearing seems to have a direct imprint on our brain. What we repeatedly hear gets imprinted. As a result we need to carefully select what we listen to and let in only what's necessary or healthy for us.

If you've ever said a bad word in front of a toddler who was learning to speak, you know the power of listening and recording. Usually it's difficult to break a child from speaking a bad word you didn't mean for him or her to hear.

Take notice of your environment throughout the day and remove any unnecessary or unpleasant noises. Is there a noise that makes you shudder? If you live in a city, maybe traffic noise is creating a disturbance in your environment. Are there too many noises in your environment? For example, there are several people who reside with me. At any given time, we could have the radio and TV going, someone playing music upstairs, and a conversation going on somewhere else. I've learned to turn off the unnecessary noise and advise others to be quieter so I can have my peace.

Replace environmental noise with pleasant sounds. Sounds of nature are almost always soothing. If you don't have nature surrounding you, or it's a cold day, play recorded music with nature sounds, such as ocean sounds, or any other pleasant musical sounds. If you live in a busy city, invest in a white-noise machine or indoor fountain so you can drown out the bustling outdoor activity. Play your soothing sounds in the office too; if you're with colleagues, use headphones to shut out the surrounding sounds.

Try silence for a day or two. When at home alone or in the car, strive to not turn on the TV or radio. Allow silence to penetrate your home. At first, you may get anxious or annoyed, especially if you're used to background noise. But soon you will find it pleasant and inviting. You will feel a sense of peace and serenity. And you will begin to crave the silence. Your mind will become clearer and your sense of intuition honed.

Touch

At first when we think of touch, it may be difficult to associate it with our environment. But touch surrounds us in all our environments. In addition to human touch, our environment is touching us all the time. Think about where you are sitting right now. Are you sitting in a couch or a comfy chair? Are you at a café drinking coffee or eating somewhere? Or perhaps you're lounging on a chair by the beach? What do you feel about the place where you're sitting while reading? Is it comfortable? Would you prefer some pillows or a blanket?

If you stop and think about it, you'll see that our clothing touches us, our furniture touches us, and the seat in our car touches us. Think about all the things throughout the day that touch you — even the keyboard on your computer!

Go through each environment you encounter daily and notice the objects surrounding you. Make a mental note of the things you don't like touching you, and see if you can do something about them. For example, there may be an uncomfortable couch that hurts your back and you never want to sit there. Or maybe your desk chair is causing you pain during your eight-hour workday. Make a list of all the things you can change in order to enhance your tactile environment.

TAKE ADVANTAGE OF HEALING TOUCH

Our environment provides us with opportunities for healing touch, which is all around us. If you have a pet, you know how good it feels to stroke your pet. It feels both amazing and therapeutic at the same time. The grass outside is nice for walking barefoot in warm weather. If you live by the beach, running barefoot in the sand provides a healing touch as it connects you to the earth. Gardening is a way to touch the earth and create something beautiful, tasty, or both. Running your hands or feet through trickling or flowing water allows your skin to be massaged effortlessly. Warming your hands by a fire or allowing its heat to penetrate your face and skin are ways to reconnect to the environmental elements, which are also a part of us.

Vata types respond best to the senses of hearing and touch. If you are predominately Vata and feeling out of balance, pay extra attention to these two senses.

Sight

With the amount of visual information we have at our disposal in the twenty-first century, it's becoming increasingly difficult to filter out visual stimuli that doesn't serve us. Each electronic device provides us with visuals at our fingertips. Just like the senses of smell and hearing, our sense of sight provides us with an instantaneous imprint on our memory. Attempt to erase a disturbing image from your past and you'll recognize that it's difficult to do. For optimal health, it's imperative that you're selective in the visual stimuli you allow into your being. Motivational speaker and author Dr. Wayne Dyer points out that, when you've heard something once, it ceases to be news. I will extend that to visual perception: when you see it once, it ceases to be news. News channels and websites tend to repeat images incessantly. A constant influx of violent and disturbing images creates stress hormones in our bodies and leaves us susceptible to illness. I made a decision long ago to no longer watch the news or movies that contain violence. When there is a choice between using my sense of sight to perceive beauty, awe, and wonder, or perceiving mental disturbance, I choose beauty. You may think it's a naive approach to life. After all, violence does exist on the planet. If we close our eyes to reality, are we also closing our eyes to change? Let me ask you this: By watching a story about murder, rape, incest, or abuse, are you making the world a better place? By holding those images in your mind, are you stopping any of the violence? Or are you simply feeling bad and frightened that the world is such a scary place? I believe the true answer is the latter. I've never known war to stop because spectators watched images of war.

Surround yourself with beauty. Notice the natural beauty that exists all around you. Make a commitment to yourself to walk away from disturbing images, which are not serving you and the greater good. Your intuition will let you know how to make that choice.

Then turn curiosity into compassion. If there is an accident scene and I'm driving by, instead of gawking at the gore, I drive by and say a prayer for those involved. If I see a homeless person in the street, I make a choice to give money or food or say a silent prayer. When you see a person in need and you can help, do so. Those are ways in which you can open your eyes to love.

Please don't get me wrong. I'm not asking you to go around blindly and pretend there are not people in need or injustices in the world. You can get this information from print media or the radio. Instead of remaining mired in the misery of the world, make a decision to go out there and do something about it. The end to violence, poverty, sadness, and misery begins with each of us. Look to your own thoughts, inner dialogue, and actions first. Heal yourself first, and then you can go out and help heal the world.

Outlining the Environments in My Daily Life

Healing your sense of sight may be extended to the physical environment surrounding you at all times. Your immediate physical environment is your bedroom, kitchen, living room, car, office space, or any other place where you spend a significant amount of time. The energy in the physical objects and space around you affects your health.

Redefining the Space That Surrounds Me

Is there a space in your home you cannot enter because it gives you a sick feeling inside? Maybe it's a table, in a particular room, piled high with clutter. Or perhaps it's a room with ugly furniture.

In Ayurveda, akasha, one of the five great elements, not only defines the concept of space but also includes the openness necessary to allow new possibilities to come into your life. For example, have you ever filled a closet with so much stuff that when you tried to add something to it, the object didn't fit inside? The lack of space, or akasha, meant there was no room for the new; this left only the accumulation of the old and, as a result, no more possibilities. We can regard this energy in relation to your sense of hospitality and allowing people into your life. Maybe you have had the experience of a disorderly and cluttered home and felt embarrassed to invite people over or have guests spontaneously arrive. Because of this lack of akasha, you blocked out the flow of abundance and new experiences into your life. The concept may seem far-reaching, but it makes complete sense. Have you ever cleaned and purged a closet and felt especially good afterward, as if you could breathe better?

Ideally, every space you occupy should give you a great feeling and a sense of abundance. It doesn't cost a lot to surround yourself with beauty in your home or office space. Plants and flowers do wonders. A few candles, along with some inexpensive art or photos of loved ones and great times, create balance and a warm, cozy feeling.

Exercise: Space-Clearing Commitment

If your physical environment is not one that nourishes you each and every day, make a commitment to get rid of all the objects that no longer serve you and to create beauty in those spaces. I am aware that this can be a daunting task if you haven't done it in a long time. A great resource I used about fifteen years ago, when I had small children at home, was FlyLady.net (www.fly lady.net/d/getting-started/). Author and leader Marla Cilley is truly a genius at teaching women (and men, of course) who, whether they stay at home or work outside the home, have a difficult time managing the demands of home. What's beautiful about Cilley's approach is that she takes you through daily tasks in baby steps, so you don't feel overwhelmed.

Take stock of the rooms or spaces in your home that need the greatest amount of attention, and make a commitment to clear these spaces within a set amount of time. Complete the following prompts.

I make a commitment to clearing:

I will create beauty in these spaces by:

The Dosha Response to Environment

According to your mind-body type, you will act and react to your environment a certain way. Your natural inclination to be neat or messy, to own a lot of material possessions or only a small number, may depend largely on your doshas. This can be refreshing to learn, so that you don't feel you have to fit into a certain mold that others may cast for you.

Vata Types

Vatas are highly creative and may be a bit messy in the home and at work. Orderliness is not necessarily at the top of their priority list. A Vata type will also move or change residences often, out of boredom or the need to be constantly on the move. However, Vata types do better in an orderly environment and are less likely to go out of balance when they have some structure. To remain in balance, a Vata type needs to put down roots somewhere and create stability. She can always cater to her creative nature by painting a room a different color every few months or buying new curtains or bedsheets to keep things fresh and new.

Earthy colors such as beige, brown, and deep shades of red tend to balance Vatas.

Pitta Types

Pittas have a tendency to be a bit obsessive-compulsive with their environments. They may be accused of being neat freaks. A healthy Pitta will enjoy a clean, orderly environment where everything is in its place. A Pitta out of balance will tend toward compulsive cleanliness or perfectionism in the home or work environment. Connecting with nature or the outdoors is important for a Pitta type to help him stay in balance. Gardening is an example of an activity that connects you to the earth and allows you to get a little dirty. It will help you remember that things don't have to be perfect all the time. If you are a Pitta living with a Vata or Kapha type, allow him a space where he can express his unique style too. Expecting a Vata to be too neat or a Kapha to get rid of all of his stuff will dissatisfy both of you.

To pacify Pitta, use cooling colors in a living or work space, such as shades of green and blue or any pastels.

Kapha Types

Since Kapha types don't enjoy change very much, they have a tendency to accumulate clutter or may even hoard. If you move the furniture around or change decor, a Kapha will feel out of sorts and may get a little upset. The water and earth elements in a Kapha cause her to hold on to things even when the objects no longer serve a purpose. Crowding rooms with too much clutter will bog a Kapha type down. If you are a Kapha who sees this pattern, have a friend come over every couple of months to help you weed out your closets or rooms to keep the energy open and flowing.

To pacify Kapha, use vibrant colors in a space, such as red and yellow.

Reconnecting to the Outer Environment: Living outside Our Boxes

I enjoy travel, especially travel to faraway places. There is nothing more humbling than traveling to another country where spaces are smaller or there aren't as many amenities as we have in the United States. Living out of a suitcase for a couple of weeks reminds me, when I come home, how big my house is and how fortunate and blessed I am to have so much abundance. Travel helps me get outside of my set of boxes.

When we get stuck in the rut of routine, we often have a difficult time seeing clearly and offering ourselves a bigger picture. We become absorbed into daily life and doing and seeing the same things day after day. When this happens, small, insignificant things become big. In order to enlarge our view, we need to vary our visual perspectives from time to time.

This is easier to do than you might think. Imagine your day, and think about how you can connect to your outer environment. It could be something big, such as taking a day off from work and heading to a beach, mountain, or lake to do absolutely nothing but contemplate life. It could also be something smaller, such as taking a completely different route to work and noticing the landscape around you. Get in the habit of infusing newness into your day.

Make it a point to appreciate nature and beauty around you and connect to it. When you begin to notice how perfectly orchestrated nature is as a result of seemingly little effort, your perspective shifts. You recognize how caught up you can get in trivial matters. Then you begin to realize that little things are not such a big deal.

As I noted earlier in the book, a box can be anything from our home to our office to our vehicle. It can also be the TV or computer. The biggest box, though, is the mental box that limits our beliefs and thinking.

Reaching out and reconnecting is more difficult today because of the conveniences of daily life. If you happen to be an introvert or a little on the shy side, it's even trickier to come out to connect. While I can be very sociable, I also have a naturally timid side. Making phone calls used to be one of my greatest fears in life. And it wasn't because I was afraid of making a call. I was always afraid of bothering people. So you can imagine how happy I was at the advent of email. But while email connects you to others, it's also a form of disconnect. Living outside the boxes we have and the boxes we build will take us outside our comfort zone. And that's actually okay, because that's how we grow.

As an experiment, at the suggestion of a teacher at my son's Montessori preschool, we did a TV-free week. There is a national campaign that used to be called TV Turn-Off Week and is now called Screen-Free Week (www.screenfree.org). When we did our TV-free week about twelve years ago, it was a difficult but enlightening task. Each day we received a hand-out from the school giving us a list of reasons why we should turn off the TV. One of the reasons that struck me as the most compelling was this: in today's society, people tend to create stronger bonds with TV characters than actual people. Now we can extend this to YouTube videos, Facebook, Instagram, Twitter, and Tumblr friends. You get the picture. Instead of going out there, living life, and creating real bonds with real people in real situations, many of us are hiding behind screens.

If you are to begin living outside your box, it will require you to step out of your comfort zone. Take a step to join an actual activity outside your home. Ask a neighbor or friend to go walking with you once or twice a week. A great way to connect to your outer environment is to volunteer your time. You can integrate an interest or hobby of yours with volunteering. Do a screen-free week on your own or with your family. Jump out of your complacency and into life. We live here, in this life, in this environment. Embrace it!

Exercise: Ways You Can Live Outside Your Boxes

In order to expand your sense of self and your environment, commit either to seeing a place once a week (or month) or to trying a new activity that doesn't involve watching TV or surfing the Internet. Much of your personal growth will come from experiencing new things. When we do this we tend to see things differently and get stimulated creatively. Our perspective also tends to change as we see life from a different angle. In the following exercise, first list where you are stuck in your own "boxes" and then list how you can expand outside of your current environments.

These are the boxes I live in (physical, mental):

Ways in which I can start living outside my boxes:

EXAMPLES: Take one day a month and travel to a new place. Ride a bike to work once a week. Join a book club or volleyball team. Invite a neighbor over for coffee. Volunteer at an animal shelter.

✔ Checklist for Health

Healing Your Environments

❏ Consider each of the five senses and determine how you can enhance your sensory environments.

❏ Complete the exercise Space-Clearing Commitment.

❏ Complete the exercise Ways You Can Live Outside Your Boxes.

❏ List ways you can create beauty in all your environments, taking into account your dominant dosha.

CHAPTER ELEVEN

BREAKING *a* SPOKE
of the WHEEL

*If we could change ourselves, the tendencies in the world would
also change. As a man changes his own nature, so does the
attitude of the world change towards him.... We need not wait
to see what others do.*

— MAHATMA GANDHI

Like riding a bike, living, too, is a balancing act. Generally,
when we focus on one area of our life, another area is lack-
ing. Maybe that part is an area of your life you've completely
ignored for a long time. For some people it's their body. For
others it's finances. Perhaps for you, it's your spiritual life or
your relationships. Whatever the case, there is always an area
for improvement and an area where we feel inadequate or ill
equipped to create progress. This is where patience comes in.

You're creating a shift in your approach to life in general.
Taking a holistic approach may seem overwhelming or even
impossible at times. It is not an easy process. You're rewiring
your brain and your body. Learn to take baby steps: take one
chapter or one spoke of the wheel at a time, practice it for a

while, and master it before moving on. Changes do not happen overnight. Processing takes time too. It may be useful to read *The Wheel of Healing with Ayurveda* a second time before attempting to carry out any of the exercises.

On a positive note, changes do tend to have a ripple effect. For example, when you start to eat better or balance your mind-body type, you will begin to crave exercise or will sleep better. Or when you manage your emotions, you may feel compelled to learn meditation or improve your relationships.

Make a decision about what you would like to change first. What is most important at this time in your life? In other words, what must change?

When I teach meditation, I always tell my students in the first ten minutes of class that if they don't practice, they won't see results. And with consistent daily practice, they will see results faster. I also share with them the information that it takes about two hundred repetitions of a newly acquired skill before it becomes a habit. Anything you're doing now that you want to change, you've been doing for a considerable amount of time, so you've had a lot of practice. If you've been eating cheeseburgers your whole life and neglecting green vegetables, you have a lot of practice eating cheeseburgers. If you've been a worrier, you don't have a lot of practice managing your emotions. Be patient with yourself as you go through this process.

Dealing with Illness
While Learning an Ayurvedic Lifestyle

Many people come to holistic health and healing because of an illness. In my own life, I remember saying to a boyfriend who was vegan and trying out a macrobiotic diet: "Hey, if I ever get cancer, I'll try a macrobiotic diet." Do you see that this logic was flawed from the get-go? My focus was not on preventive health; rather, I saw Ayurvedic health care as a tool to use once I got sick. That said, if you are dealing with a chronic or acute illness, or you are experiencing symptoms but don't yet have a diagnosis, you can use Ayurvedic health care in conjunction with conventional medicine.

In fact, when I was diagnosed with cancer, I did a fair amount of research on the vegan diet and different modalities of complementary and alternative medicine. While I still went the traditional route (following allopathic recommendations), I was able to integrate a vegan diet, ate only organic foods, and drank distilled water and herbal teas.

Ayurvedic medicine does not suggest following a vegan diet; but a mostly vegetarian diet is helpful in any case. When you are ill, not only are you out of balance but also your body is depleted of the vital energy it needs to repair cells. The more you give it whole organic foods with antioxidants, phytochemicals, and vitamins, the easier it will be for your body to heal. The way I look at it is this: if you bought a Ferrari and the manufacturer suggested premium high-octane gasoline, and you gave it only regular unleaded, it might run, but poorly. The same goes for your body. If you give it some vegetables and a little fruit, and you get your calories mainly from other sources, your body will run, but not as well as it would if you gave it a lot of fresh vegetables and fresh fruit.

The great part of living an Ayurvedic lifestyle is that it's gentle on the body. So even if you're undergoing surgery, chemotherapy, or radiation, or you take prescription medications, you can also try all the methods outlined in this book, which treat the body kindly.

Healing from Addictions

Addictions are simply disconnects from your true nature. They are a search for pleasure in a vast pool of pain. Addiction means turning to an object for your pleasure rather than turning to your higher self or spiritual self for bliss. We can be addicted to most anything, from alcohol or drugs to excessive Internet use.

Disengaging from a strong addiction to a substance generally requires professional care until the substance has been purged from the body and any withdrawal symptoms have subsided. If you have a problem with substances such as alcohol or recreational or prescription drugs, I suggest seeking medical and professional help before applying the principles in this book. Once you're on the road to recovery, you can begin making use of *The Wheel of Healing*, which will in turn help you create wholeness in your body, mind, soul, and spirit so that cravings for the object of addiction are less likely to return.

If your addiction is not substance related, or it is an addiction to a lesser mind-altering substance, such as tobacco, then you can begin working on the aspects of the wheel. The more you connect to your spiritual self through the practice of meditation and expanded awareness, the less you will need the object you crave. One way you can begin to decrease usage of the object of addiction is through awareness and association. An addictive habit may be just that, a habit — a habit that has spiraled out of control and turned into an obsession. Habits tend to share similar patterns. We perform them under certain circumstances and with certain associations. For example, if you are a smoker, perhaps you've always had a cigarette with your morning coffee in the kitchen. The associative behaviors are drinking coffee and sitting in the kitchen. If you take away the associative behaviors, you are breaking a pattern. If you are a smoker with this particular association, I suggest that you have the morning cigarette in a place you would normally never associate with smoking, such as in the bathtub or in a room of the house you rarely go to. Then, you would consume the cigarette consciously. Focus only on smoking and sensations in the body, rather than on any distractions. In this way, you are creating new neuroassociations with smoking.

The same can go for overeating. People who overeat tend to have triggers. Perhaps one trigger is watching TV late at night. A person who munches in front of the TV late at night might instead take his snack to the table in the dining room, set out a nice place mat, and focus consciously on the same food. Again, it's about breaking the pattern and creating a new pattern, but with total awareness of the behavior.

The more you heal the body and mind and connect with your spiritual self, the less your addictions can maintain a grip on you. Know that healing is possible, and that the essence of who you are is stronger than any addiction.

What If You Get Stuck on One Spoke and Cannot Move On?

Often when we pick up a self-help book, we come to it for a reason. Our physical health is poor or our emotions are a wreck. Maybe we're in a life transition or looking for our life's purpose. Whatever compelled you to pick up this book, you're here. So you began reading or working on a section. And once you began, you found that self-improvement is not easy. Then you got stuck, mired deeply in the problem that prompted you to purchase the book in the first place. Frustrated, you now fear you cannot move on to the other sections.

Let me assure you, nothing could be farther from the truth. Have you ever, in your life, taken a standardized test? Or any timed test at all? What do all test strategists recommend? Work on the easy questions first, putting a small mark on the difficult ones; then, at the end, you can go back to the tricky ones. Success is a better motivator than frustration. We are ever evolving and ever changing. There is always room to grow, even in the areas where you believe you don't need improvement. In fact, begin the work with your strongest aspect of health, tweak it, and then move on to your second strongest.

Staying stuck will get you nowhere. Life is not perfect. It's naturally rather messy. Keep the wheel moving, and soon you will find you're rolling smoothly. You'll see new scenery, experience greater landscapes, and see the world before you in all its infinite possibilities.

CHAPTER TWELVE

ROLLING SMOOTHLY

Enjoying the Ride

You have to distinguish yourself and operate at the highest level of ethics, of integrity, of veracity. If you lower yourself to the level of a lot of the people in the world today, you won't be distinctive. You won't be preeminent. You won't stand out.

— JAY ABRAHAM

Most of life is a process. The lessons we learn are part of the journey, not the outcome. Know that outcomes are okay, but they simply set us up for more processes.

Karmic Action: Doing What's Right

Living an Ayurvedic lifestyle includes performing right action. The word *karma* literally means action. The essence of karma is found in the timeless saying "What goes around comes around." At first glance, this appears to be negative. We've all heard people say, "You'll get what's coming to you." In my own upbringing I heard phrases such as "God will punish you."

The true meaning of karma goes beyond punishment by

an outside source. It's accountability for your actions in every moment. Jay Abraham, who in my opinion is an absolute genius in business and marketing, has explained the meaning of integrity. Abraham teaches that in order to measure a man's integrity, look at how he behaves when things aren't going well, as opposed to how he behaves when things *are* going well. A man with integrity will act even better when things are not going well.

It is my observation that in today's world, not many people have integrity in the truest sense. How do you act when no one is looking? How do you behave when you are accountable to no one but yourself? Living up to the highest moral standards lets you live in optimal health. If you are not convinced of this statement, look at the health of someone who lies frequently. Or observe someone who takes advantage of others, and notice how healthy he or she is.

Karma is choosing spontaneous right action in every moment of every day for your entire life. How is that for accountability? Does it seem heavy? Well, it is. But it's not as difficult as you may think. Do you personally know anyone who lives by such standards? What kind of person is he or she? Do you respect this person immensely? You may ask, "How do I know what action is spontaneously right?" The answer is: you know. You know more than you believe you know. Your body knows, your mind and your soul know.

The best way to roll smoothly through all the spokes of the wheel and make your wheel whole is to observe the choices you make in each moment. You will feel in your body whether a decision is right or wrong for you. If it's wrong, your heart will beat faster, you will get a sinking feeling in your stomach, or your inner voice will tell you not to do it. This applies to any decision you need to make, from deciding whether to eat a piece of cake to deciding whether to spend money. Always pause and notice how your body feels. Your body has an innate intelligence beyond what you can imagine.

In the beginning, you may resist making correct choices because you're accustomed to overriding this natural intelligence. But with practice, you will begin to live a karmic life. It's a responsible life, one that doesn't leave a lot of room for error.

So what is the payoff? The payoff is your inner peace. The payoff is knowing that you're doing the right thing rather than merely the easy thing. Anyone can do what is easy, and most of us do. But few people consistently do what is right.

When you begin to live this way, things naturally run smoothly for you. The universe has a way of rewarding karmically correct behavior. The rewards come because you are acting in accordance with universal laws. And when you live according to universal laws, the road opens wide and few obstacles lie ahead.

On Being Gentle, Humble, Loving, and Kind

You are on a beautiful path, one that will take you not only to health and healing but also to a more meaningful life. Something brought you to this path and urged you to try it out. It's normal to be excited and enthusiastic and sometimes a bit zealous. But know that not everyone is on this path yet, and some may never be. Changes and self-improvement take us to higher heights and different dimensions. At times these roads can seem lonely. We want so much for our loved ones to join us on this journey to wellness and a life of expanded awareness. You may even feel disconnected from the ones you love as you begin to heal. Know that this is normal. There doesn't have to be disconnect. You can approach your loved ones with compassion and kindness. A sense of arrogance may try to take over as you heal — your ego and mind may think you're better or more advanced than others around you. But let your heart open up instead, and be an example for the people in your life. Let the light of your expanded awareness shine for others to see. In time, they will be attracted to the light and will wonder what you're doing differently. With a smile you can explain how you're now living and what you are doing. But do it with humility.

Celebrate the new you and your commitment to wholeness. I wish you the best on your journey and many blessings for years to come.

Om stamanam bhavatu satayuh
purusah satendriya ayusyevendriye prati tisthati.
(May your life measure a hundred years.
May your sense organs be healthy for a hundred years,
and may the spirit remain in your life and sense organs.)

— YAJUR VEDA, TAITTIRIYA SAMHITA 2.3.11

SUN SALUTATIONS (SURYA NAMASKAR)

The Sun Salutations are a series of yoga poses that lengthen and strengthen every major muscle group in the body. Each Sun Salutation provides flexibility and strength. When done in cycles over a twenty-minute period, the series can provide cardiovascular exercise as well. Follow the photo illustrations to learn and practice the Sun Salutations daily.

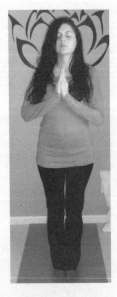 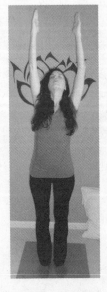 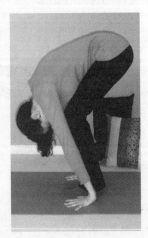

1. Salutation Pose   2. Sky-Reaching Pose   3. Hand-to-Foot Pose

1. SALUTATION POSE

Begin with the feet parallel and big toes touching; bring your hands to your heart center and close your eyes. Take a cleansing breath through the nose. Hold gratitude in your heart and set an intention for your practice.

2. SKY-REACHING POSE

Bring your arms down, around, and up, taking a slight backbend, and gaze toward the sky as you inhale.

3. HAND-TO-FOOT POSE

Exhale and swan dive forward, bringing your arms out to the sides. Align hands with the toes. If you need to, bend your knees a little to bring your palms flat on the mat.

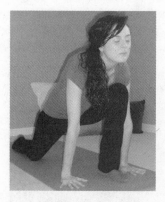

4. Equestrian Pose

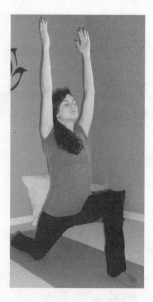

5. Sky Reaching in
Equestrian Pose

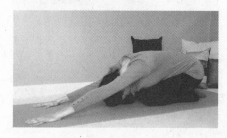

6. Child's Pose (First Variation)

4. EQUESTRIAN POSE

Take your right foot back in a lunge and place both hands beside your front foot. Make sure your knee is aligned with the ankle.

5. SKY REACHING IN EQUESTRIAN POSE

From the equestrian pose, reach both arms up overhead as you inhale and gaze slightly upward.

6. CHILD'S POSE (FIRST VARIATION)

Bring your hands back to the floor, bring the front foot back, and sit on your heels.

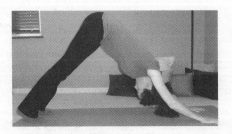

7. Down Dog (Second Variation)

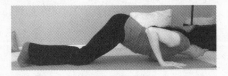

8. Eight Limbs Pose

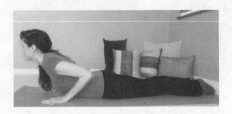

9. Cobra Pose

7. Down Dog (Second Variation)

From the equestrian pose, take one foot back and lift your body into an inverted letter *V*, with your tailbone reaching into the air and chest approaching the thighs. Feet are hip-width apart, and hands are shoulder-width apart. Your weight is over the feet rather than over the hands.

8. Eight Limbs Pose

Lower your knees, bend your elbows toward your hips, and bring your chest and chin toward the floor. Hands are aligned with the shoulders.

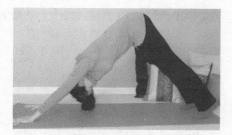

10. Down Dog or Child's Pose

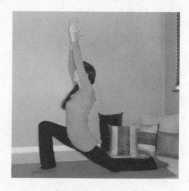

11. Equestrian Pose

9. COBRA POSE

Flatten out on your belly. Bring your fingertips into alignment with your shoulders. Bring your elbows in toward the torso. Elongate your legs, with the feet touching each other. Lift your chest and face up while keeping your feet on the floor.

10. DOWN DOG OR CHILD'S POSE

Push back into either the child's pose or down dog.

11. EQUESTRIAN POSE

Bring your right foot forward and place your hands on either side of the right foot. The back leg is elongated and the knee is on the floor.

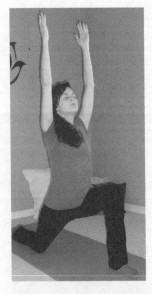

12. Equestrian Sky Reaching

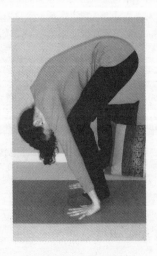

13. Hand-to-Foot Pose

12. Equestrian Sky Reaching

In equestrian pose, bring both arms up overhead as you inhale.

13. Hand-to-Foot Pose

Bring the left foot forward and place both hands alongside the feet. Bow your head forward toward your knees as you exhale.

14. Sky-Reaching Pose

Reach both arms up overhead, and let your palms touch as you inhale. Gaze up toward the sky.

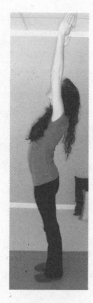

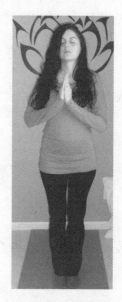

14. Sky-Reaching Pose

15. Salutation Pose

15. Salutation Pose

Exhale and bring your hands to your heart.

Repeat on the other side, starting with the left leg back, in the equestrian pose. Beginners, start with three sets, and as you advance try to do six or twelve sets.

NOTES

Introduction: Reinventing the Wheel?

1. Division of Nutrition, Physical Activity, and Obesity, National Center for Chronic Disease Prevention and Health Promotion, "Adult Overweight and Obesity," Centers for Disease Control and Prevention, last updated April 27, 2012, www.cdc.gov/obesity/adult/index.html. The study was conducted in 2010.
2. National Center for Chronic Disease Prevention and Health Promotion, "Chronic Diseases: The Leading Causes of Death and Disability in the United States," Centers for Disease Control and Prevention, last updated May 9, 2014, www.cdc.gov/chronicdisease/overview/index.htm.
3. Ibid.

Chapter 2. The Entire Wheel

1. "Pet Benefit Articles and Information," Pets for the Elderly Foundation, undated, accessed November 4, 2014, www.petsfortheelderly.org/articles.html.
2. "Diana Nyad," *Bio*, A&E Television Networks, December 9, 2014, www.biography.com/people/diana-nyad-21329683#synopsis.

Chapter 3. Physical Health

1. "Global Cancer Rates Could Increase by 50% to 15 million by 2020," World Health Organization, April 3, 2003, www.who.int/mediacentre/news/releases/2003/pr27/en/.
2. "Overweight and Obesity: Data and Statistics," Centers for Disease Control and Prevention, last updated September 9, 2014, www.cdc.gov/obesity/data/index.html.

Chapter 4. Spiritual Health

1. Norwegian University of Science and Technology, "Brain Waves and Meditation," AlphaGalileo, March 19, 2010, news release, www.alphagalileo.org /ViewItem.aspx?ItemId=70952&CultureCode=en.
2. Angela Eksteins, "Meditation May Be the Future of Anti-Aging, Part I," Natural News: Natural Health News and Scientific Discoveries, February 14, 2010, www.naturalnews.com/028157_meditation_longevity.html#ixz z2UtkbiTux.
3. James Gorman, "Scientists Hint at Why Laughter Feels So Good," *New York Times*, September 13, 2011, www.nytimes.com/2011/09/14/science /14laughter.html?_r=0.

Chapter 7. Relationship Health

1. Mother Teresa, *A Simple Path* (New York: Random House, 2007), p. 79.
2. Marshall B. Rosenberg, *Nonviolent Communication: A Language of Life* (Encinitas, CA: Puddledancer Press, 2005).

Chapter 8. Occupational Health

1. Reported in "Workplace Stress," American Institute of Stress, undated, accessed November 14, 2014, www.stress.org/workplace-stress/.
2. "Work Stress on the Rise: 8 in 10 Americans Are Stressed about Their Jobs, Survey Finds," *Huffington Post*, updated April 12, 2013, www.huffington post.com/2013/04/10/work-stress-jobs-americans_n_3053428.html.
3. "Work Environment May Put Women at Risk of Diabetes," *Journal of Occupational Medicine*, Institute for Work and Health, August 21, 2012, www.iwh.on.ca/media/2012-aug-21.

Chapter 9. Financial Health

1. "American Household Credit Card Debt Statistics: 2014," NerdWallet Finance, November 2014, www.nerdwallet.com/blog/credit-card-data /average-credit-card-debt-household/.
2. "U.S. Consumer Debt Statistics 2012," Visual.ly, January 8, 2013, http://visual.ly/us-consumer-debt-statistics-and-trends-2012.

GLOSSARY *of* SANSKRIT TERMS

ABHYANGA: Daily oil massage.

AKASHA: Space or ether.

AMA: A toxic residue caused by undigested food, experiences, and emotions. The term translates as "toxins in the body and mind."

ARTHA: Material wealth, gain, or prosperity. One of the four goals in life that are known, in Vedic morality, as the *purusharthas*.

ASANA: A yoga pose.

AYURVEDA: The science of life; the name is derived from the Sanskrit words *ayus*, meaning "life," and *veda*, meaning "science or knowledge."

CHAKRAS: The energy centers in the body, related to the nerve plexus centers. There are seven main chakras, which together align the spine.

CHARAKA SAMHITA: An early text on Ayurveda. *The Charaka Samhita* and the *Sushruta Samhita* are the two foundational texts of this field; both date to the early centuries of the common era.

DHARMA: An individual's purpose in life.

DOSHA: The three main psychophysiological principles of the body (Vata, Pitta, Kapha), which determine a person's individual mind-body constitution.

244 The Wheel of Healing with Ayurveda

GHEE: Clarified butter.

JALA: Water.

KAPHA: One of the three doshas, it combines the elements water and earth. It is responsible for bodily structure.

KARMA: Action or deed. It is also the principle of causality, in which a person's intent in taking an action in the present equals a particular result in the future.

MAHABHUTAS: The great elements: space, air, fire, water, and earth.

MANTRA: Derived from two Sanskrit words: *man*, meaning "mind," and *tra*, meaning "instrument." This instrument of the mind is a sound or series of sounds used to connect body, mind, and spirit.

NASYA: Method of administering oil or herbalized oil to the nostrils. It is one of the five parts of *panchakarma*.

OJAS: Healing chemicals in the body that are by-products of properly digested food, emotions, and experiences.

PITTA: The biological humor in Ayurveda composed of the elements fire and water.

PRAKRUTI: The biological constitution of an individual. It is determined at conception and is composed of certain proportions of the three doshas: Vata, Pitta, and Kapha.

PRANA: Vital life energy, or life force.

PRANAYAMA: Yogic breathing techniques; also, the fourth branch of yoga.

PRITHIVI: The earth element.

RISHIS: Ancient sages, or seers, from India.

SURYA NAMASKAR: Sun Salutations, a series of yoga poses that coordinate with the breath.

TEJAS: Fire.

VATA: Composed of space and air, this is one of the three doshas, or Ayurvedic mind-body types.

VAYU: Wind or air.

VIKRUTI: The current state of an individual, in contrast to a person's natural state, or *prakruti*. This state may indicate imbalances in an individual's mind-body constitution.

YOGA: Derived from the Sanskrit word *yuj*, which means "to yoke" or "to join together." In yoga, we join together our mind, body, soul, and spirit.

RECOMMENDED WEBSITES
and AYURVEDIC RESOURCES

THE AYURVEDIC PATH: www.theayurvedicpath.com. Michelle
  Fondin's yoga and health studio in Herndon, Virginia.
THE CHOPRA CENTER FOR WELLBEING: www.chopra.com/.
  Ayurvedic products and workshops.
CHOPRA CENTER TEACHERS: www.choprateachers.com/. Find
  a Primordial Sound Meditation teacher in your area.
FIND A FOOD CO-OP: www.localharvest.org/organic-farms/.
FLYLADY.NET: www.flylady.net/. Find help in getting your
  home and life in order using daily task reminders and
  motivation.
MAHARISHI AYURVEDIC PRODUCTS INTERNATIONAL:
  www.mapi.com/. Ayurvedic products.
NATURAL BY NATURE GRASS-FED DAIRY PRODUCTS:
  www.natural-by-nature.com/.

REFERENCES *and* RECOMMENDED READING

Buscaglia, Leo. *Love.* New York: Fawcett Books, 1972.

Chapman, Gary. *The 5 Love Languages: The Secret to Love That Lasts.* Chicago: Northfield, 2010.

Chopra, Deepak. *Magical Mind, Magical Body.* Simon and Schuster Audio / Nightingale-Conant, 2003.

———. *Perfect Health: The Complete Mind/Body Guide.* New York: Harmony Books, 1991.

———. *The Spontaneous Fulfillment of Desire: Harnessing the Infinite Power of Coincidence.* New York: Three Rivers Press, 2003.

Chopra, Deepak, and David Simon. *The Seven Spiritual Laws of Yoga.* Hoboken, NJ: John Wiley and Sons, 2005.

Dyer, Wayne W. *The Power of Intention: Learning to Co-create Your World Your Way.* Carlsbad, CA: Hay House, 2005.

Edelman, Ric. *The Truth about Money.* 4th ed. New York: Harper Business, 2010.

Goleman, Daniel. *Emotional Intelligence.* New York: Random House, 1995.

Gray, John. *Mars and Venus Together Forever: Relationship Skills for Lasting Love.* New York: Harper Perennial, 2005.

Harley, Willard F., Jr. *Fall in Love, Stay in Love.* Grand Rapids, MI: Revell Books, 2001.

———. *His Needs, Her Needs: Building an Affair-Proof Marriage.* Grand Rapids, MI: Revell Books, 2011.

Iyengar, B. K. S. *Light on Life: The Yoga Journey to Wholeness, Inner Peace, and Ultimate Freedom.* Emmaus, PA: Rodale Press, 2005.

Johari, Harish. *Chakras: Energy Centers of Transformation.* Rochester, VT: Destiny Books, 2000.

Judith, Anodea. *Wheels of Life.* St. Paul, MN: Llewellyn, 1994.

Lad, Vasant. *Textbook of Ayurveda: Fundamental Principles.* Vol. 1. Albuquerque, NM: Ayurvedic Press, 2002.

Morningstar, Amadea. *Ayurvedic Cooking for Westerners: Familiar Western Food Prepared with Ayurvedic Principles.* Twin Lakes, WI: Lotus Press, 1995.

Orman, Suze. *The 9 Steps to Financial Freedom.* New York: Crown, 2006.

————. *Women and Money: Owning the Power to Control Your Destiny.* New York: Spiegel and Grau, 2007.

Pollan, Michael. *In Defense of Food: An Eater's Manifesto.* New York: Penguin, 2009.

————. *Omnivore's Dilemma: A Natural History of Four Meals.* New York: Penguin, 2006.

Rosenberg, Marshall. *Nonviolent Communication: A Language of Life.* Encinitas, CA: Puddledancer Press, 2005.

Simon, David. *Vital Energy: The 7 Keys to Invigorate Body, Mind and Soul.* New York: John Wiley and Sons, 2000.

Simon, David, and Deepak Chopra. *The Wisdom of Healing.* New York: Three Rivers Press, 1997.

Tirtha, Sadashiva. *The Ayurveda Encyclopedia: Natural Secrets to Healing, Prevention and Longevity.* Unadilla, NY: Ayurveda Holistic Center Press, 2007.

Weil, Andrew. *8 Weeks to Optimum Health.* New York: Ballantine, 1997.

INDEX

Abraham, Jay, 229, 230
acceptance, 160, 167
accumulation (disease stage), 26
acid reflux, 144
action(s): right, 107–12, 229–31; taking responsibility for, 162–63
addictions, 143, 226–27
advertising, 50, 71
aggravation (disease stage), 26
aging, premature, 67
air (*vayu*), 15, 76
alcohol, avoidance of, 83–84
alienation, 147
American Heart Association, 50
anger, 116
anorexia, 142
antioxidants, 67
anxiety, 116, 142, 154
apathy, 147
apologies, 168
aromatherapy, 84
arrogance, 232
artha (wealth), 153, 196–97
arthritis, 142
asthma, 145
astringent (food taste type), 62, 65, 77–78

atheism, 94
awareness, witnessing, 99–101, 107
awe, experiencing, 109
Ayurveda: author's experience, xvii–xix, 7; as balanced healing approach, xviii, 13, 223; checklist for, 32; daily practice of, 224; defined, 11–13; environment as extended body in, 207–8; food tastes in, 61–66, 64–65; glossary, 243–45; health as defined in, 13–14; humility and, 231–32; inward direction of, 7; *mahabhutas* (great elements), 14–15; mind-body type in, 8; physician consultations in, 31; problems encountered while practicing, 223–28; reasons for following, 12–13; right action and, 229–31; symptom plans in, 31–32; Vedanta as origin of, 135; Western medicine vs., 28–29; wheel as analogy for, xx, 5–6, 223–24; wholeness principle in, 3–5, 12, 158, 232. *See also* doshas (mind-body types)
Ayurvedic Mind-Body Type Test, 15–22

Ayurvedic nutrition plan, 57–70,
    91–92; dosha-specific diets, 74–79;
    exercises, 78–79; food tastes in,
    61–66, 209; freshly prepared
    foods, 59–60; 90-10 rule in, 58, 70;
    organic foods, 60–61, 66–68, 209;
    sample meals, 66; *sattvic* (healing)
    foods, 66–67; unhealthy foods
    reduced/eliminated in, 67–69;
    water in, 69–70
Ayurvedic Path Yoga studio, 88, 102,
    186

baths, 85–86
bhastrika breath, 144
bitter (food taste type), 62, 65, 77–78
bladder problems, 143
blame, 162–63, 168
blood pressure, 145, 196
boat pose, 144
body: extended, environment as,
    207–8; intuition and sensations in,
    96–97; meditation effects upon,
    102–3; as sacred, 54; self-love of, 152
boredom, 147
bound angle pose, 143
bow pose, 144
breathing: alternate-nostril, 147;
    bhastrika breath, 144; for creative/
    sexual chakra (*svadhisthana*),
    143–44; *kapalabati* ("skull-shining
    breath"), 144; *ujjayi* yogic breath-
    ing technique, 146
bridge pose, 146
Buddha, 33
Buscaglia, Leo, 110, 151, 159
butter, organic, 67–68

caffeine, avoidance of, 83–84
calories, 59
camel pose, 145
cancer: author's experience, xvii–xix,
    139–40; diet and prevention of, 67;
    US rates of, 1
candles, 216
cardiovascular training, 87–88
car loans, 202
chakras: author's experience, 139–40;
    creative/sexual (*svadhisthana*),
    143–44; crown (*sahaswara*), 147–48;
    defined, 139; heart (*anahata*),
    144–45; root (*muladhara*), 142–43;
    solar plexus (*manipura*), 144;
    third-eye (*ajna*), 146–47; throat
    (*vishuddha*), 145–46; unblocking,
    139–42
Charaka Samhita, 11, 12, 30
checklists for health: Ayurveda, 32;
    dharma (life's purpose), 48; emo-
    tional health, 130; environmental
    health, 222; financial health, 206;
    occupational health, 193; the past,
    149; physical health, 91–92; relation-
    ship health, 180–81; spirituality/
    spiritual health, 112
chemotherapy, 225
child's pose, 147, 235–36, 237
choice, conscious: conditioned
    choice vs., 98–99, 112; of emotions,
    120–22; lessons from the past and,
    137–38; relationship health and,
    176; in right action, 229–31
Chopra, Deepak, xviii, xix, 62, 94
Chopra Center, 102
Cilley, Marla, 216–17
clairvoyance, 146

clutter, 215–17, 218–19, 222

cobra pose, 143, 236, 237

colds, 146

communication: electronic, 171; about
    money, 204–5

communication skills: for relation-
    ships, 156, 163–65, 169, 170–73, 180;
    throat chakra as source of, 145

compassion, 145, 155, 170–73, 180,
    214–15, 231–32

computers, 208

concentration problems, 147

Confucius, 183

confusion, 147

constipation, 142

constitution types. *See* doshas (mind-
    body types)

co-ops, 60–61

Costco Wholesale, 56

cow face pose, 145

Creating a Plan for Transforming
    Your Current Job or Finding Your
    Ideal Job (exercise), 192–93

Creating Your Physical Movement
    Plan (exercise), 90–91

creative/sexual chakra (*svadhisthana*),
    143–44

creativity, 124

credit card debt, 196, 202

crown chakra (*sahaswara*), 147–48

dairy products, organic, 61

dance, 124

darkness, for sleep, 86, 209

dating, 178–80

Davenport, Rita, 195

debt, 196, 201, 202–3, 206

decluttering, 215–17, 222

delta waves, 107

depression, 116, 147, 154

desires, list of, 44–47

detoxification, Ayurveda and, 12

dharma (life's purpose), 5; check-
    list for, 48; defined, 35–39, 188;
    exercises, 40–41, 47; finding, 33–34,
    39–44; importance of, 34–35; in
    Indian tradition, 36, 42; intentions
    /desires list for, 44–47; as life
    category, 153; occupational health
    and, 186–89

diabetes, 66–67, 144, 183

diet: Ayurveda and, 12, 49; fat-free,
    7–8, 67–68; flexibility in, 58; Kapha-
    pacifying, 66–67; Kapha-specific,
    78; Pitta-pacifying, 66; Pitta-
    specific, 77; Vata-pacifying, 66;
    Vata-specific, 76–77; vegan, 224–25

Discovering Dharma (exercise), 40–41

disease: during Ayurvedic practice,
    224–25; chronic, in U.S., 1–2;
    dharma and, 34–35; food quality
    and, 51; six stages of, 26–28

disruption (disease stage), 27

dissemination (disease stage), 26–27

distractions, 104, 110, 170, 171

divorce, 157

dolphin pose, 147

doshas (mind-body types): diets
    tailored to, 74–79; emotional
    rebalancing specific to, 123–27, 130;
    environmental health and, 213,
    217–19, 222; financial health and,
    197; interpreting, 25–27; Kapha

doshas (mind-body types) (*continued*)
(earth principle), 24–25; occupational health and, 189–92; physical
exercise routines specific to, 89–91;
Pitta (fire principle), 23–24; plan
for balancing, 31; relationship
health and, 173–76, 181; routines
governed by, 81–83; symptom
plans for, 31–32; test for determining, 15–22; three principle types, 15;
Vata (wind principle), 22–23. *See
also specific mind-body type*
down dog pose, 236, 237
Dunbar, Robin, 109–10
Dyer, Wayne, 214

eagle's pose, 147
earth (*prithivi*), 15, 76, 142
eating, as sacred act, 79–80
eating awareness, guidelines for,
71–74, 82, 91–92, 209
Edelman, Ric, 202–3
ego, 144
eight limbs pose, 236
8 Weeks to Optimum Health (Weil),
208
Einstein, Albert, 207
elements. *See mahabhutas* (great
elements)
email, 171, 220
emotional health: checklist for, 130;
dosha-specific rebalancing for,
123–27, 130; emotional control and,
115–16, 130; exercises, 127–30; financial health and, 196; physical health
and, 113–14; tools for establishing,
116–23

Emotional Intelligence (Goleman), 118
emotional toxins, 116–17
emotional triggers, 122–23, 227
emotions: conscious choices regarding, 120–22; control over, 115–16,
130; gender differences, 115; iden-
tifying, 120, 172–73; ignoring, 119;
taking responsibility for, 118–20,
130
empathy, 145
employment. *See* jobs; occupational
health
endorphins, 110
energy: meditation as connection to,
105–6; money as, 196–97, 199–202
energy work, Ayurveda and, 12
environment: daily, redefining, 215–17;
as extended body, 207–8; for meals,
72, 73
environmental health: Ayurvedic
background of, 207–8; checklist
for, 222; doshas and, 213, 217–19,
222; exercises, 216–17, 221; natural
reconnection for, 219–21, 222;
sensory input for, 208–15, 222;
space-clearing for, 215–17, 222
envy, 143
equestrian pose, 235, 237
equestrian sky reaching pose, 235, 238
Erikson, Erik, 140
exercise, physical: Ayurveda and,
49; cardiovascular, 86, 87–88;
dosha-specific routines, 89–91;
fitness programs, 87–89; flexibility
training, 87, 88–89; importance
of, 86–87; physical health and, 51;
planning for, 57; resistance, 87;

routines for, 81–82, 92; in rural
    areas, 55
exercises: Ayurveda, 32; Ayurvedic
    nutrition plan, 78–79; dharma, 40–
    41, 47; emotional health, 127–30;
    environmental health, 216–17,
    221; financial health, 198–99, 201;
    health, 9; occupational health,
    192–93; the past, 133, 134, 148;
    physical health, 90–91; relation-
    ship health, 166–69; spirituality
    /spiritual health, 101
experimentation, 97–99
eye problems, 147

Facebook, 220
farmers' markets, 60
fatigue, physical health and, 57
fear, 142
financial health: beliefs about money
    and, 197–99, 206; checklist for, 206;
    debt reduction for, 202–3, 206;
    dosha effects on, 197; education
    about, 206; emotional health and,
    196; exercises, 198–99, 201; generos-
    ity for, 199–202, 206; gratitude for,
    199, 206; importance of, 195–96;
    physical health and, 196–97, 206;
    wealth creation for, 204–6. *See also*
    money; occupational health
fire (*tejas*), 15, 76
fish pose, 145
fitness programs, 87–89
flexibility training, 87, 88–89
flour, organic, 68
flow, 36–37
flowers, 208, 210, 216

FlyLady.net, 216–17
food: Ayurvedic taste types, 61–66;
    enjoyment of, 73; freshly prepared,
    59–60; frozen/canned, 68–69;
    locally-grown, 60–61, 209; mind-
    body connection with, 70–74;
    online sources, 56; organic, 50,
    55–56, 60–61, 66, 92, 209; portion
    control, 72; processed, 51, 66, 71,
    91; quality of, and health, 49–52,
    71; as sacred, 79–80; smell of, in
    environment, 210
food co-ops, 60–61
forgiveness, 45, 111–12
fork, putting down, 72
forward folds, 148
fountains, indoor, 212
fruit, 66–67
frustration, 227–28
fun-money budget, 205–6
future, lessons from the past taken to,
    148, 149

gallbladder disease, 51
Gandhi, Mahatma, 223
generosity, 199–202, 206, 214–15
Goleman, Daniel, 113, 118
gratitude, 45; for financial health, 199,
    206; for food, 74; heart chakra as
    source of, 145; practicing, for spiri-
    tual health, 107–8; in relationships,
    165–66, 169
gratitude journal, 108
Gray, John, 162
greed, 142
guilt, 116, 162–63, 168
"gushing," 161, 167–68

habits, addictive, 226–27
hallucinations, 147
handstands, 148
hand-to-foot pose, 234, 238
Harley, Willard, 161
hatha yoga, 88–89
headaches, 147
headstands, 148
healing: dharma and, 34–35; *sattvic* (healing) foods, 66–67
healing touch, 213
health: Ayurvedic definition of, 13–14; Ayurvedic medicine and, 7; exercises, 9; personal control over, 2, 3; responsibility shifting for, 2–3; taking back, 6–8; taking responsibility for, 8–9. *See also* emotional health; environmental health; financial health; occupational health; physical health; relationship health; spirituality/spiritual health
health care, cost of, 2
health insurance, 2, 29
hearing, sense of, 211–12
hearing problems, 146
heart attacks, 113–14, 183
heart chakra (*anahata*), 144–45
heart disease, 1, 51, 67, 145
hemorrhoids, 142
herbal medicine, 52; Ayurveda and, 12
herbal teas, 84
high-fructose corn syrup, 68, 91
Hippocrates, 49
hip swaying, 143
His Needs, Her Needs (Harley), 161
holistic approach, 223–24
honesty, 45

honey, 66–67
hopelessness, 116
Horizon Organic Dairy, 50, 61
Hugo, Victor, 126
hugs, 110–11, 167
hum (mantra), 146
humility, 231–32
hunger, eating and, 71–72
hypertension, 51
hypoglycemia, 144

immune disorders, 196
impatience, 116, 137–38, 224
inclined plane pose, 144
India, 198
Indian tradition, dharma in, 36, 42
infidelity, 156
inner voice, listening to, 97–99, 200
insecurity, 142
Instagram, 220
integrity, 45, 230
intentions, list of, 44–47
interconnectedness, 42, 155
interdependence, 155
internal dialogue, listening to, 100–101, 112
Internal-Dialogue Assessment (exercise), 101
International Journal of Neuroscience, 107
interruptions, 165
introversion, 220
intuition, 96–97, 107, 112

jealousy, 143
jobs: as dharma, 186–89; dissatisfaction with, 183–84; ideal, finding

(exercise), 192–93; learning to love, 184–85; meaning in, 185–87; moonlighting, 187; new, searching for, 185; physical/emotional health connection and, 113–14; stress related to, 183–84

journaling, 85, 108, 124

kama (desire/marriage), 153, 154

kapalabati ("skull-shining breath"), 144

Kapha dosha (earth principle) / Kapha types, 24–25; eating awareness guidelines for, 72; emotional rebalancing specific to, 127; environmental health for, 218–19; financial health and, 197; imbalances in, 75, 126–27, 155, 176; occupational health for, 191–92; physical exercise routines specific to, 90; relationship health and, 175–76; symptom plans for, 31

Kapha-pacifying diet, 66–67

Kapha-specific diet, 78

Kapha times, 81–83

karma, 229–31

kidney problems, 143

kindness: healing and, 231–32; internal dialogue and, 101; to oneself, 152; random acts of, 111; speech and, 165

kissing, 167

knee problems, 142

knee-to-chest pose, 143

knee-to-ear pose, 146

Kraft Foods, 50

lam (mantra), 143

laughter, 109–10, 162, 168

laziness, physical health and, 55–56

letter writing, 124

lifestyle: Ayurveda and, 12; "box," 109, 220–21; as illness cause, 2, 51

List of Intentions and Desires (exercise), 47

lizard pose, 143

localization (disease stage), 27

love, 45, 112, 145, 155, 159–60, 167. *See also* self-love

lovemaking, 167

lung disease, 145

macrobiotic diet, 224–25

Magical Mind, Magical Body (Chopra), 62

mahabhutas (great elements), 14–15

malpractice insurance, 29

manifestation (disease stage), 27

mantras, 102, 105; for root chakra (*muladhara*), 143

Mars and Venus Together Forever (Gray), 162

Maslow, Abraham, 37

massage therapy, 12

mates, searching for, 157–59, 178–80, 181

Matthew, Gospel of, 126

meditation: Ayurveda and, 12; benefits of, 102–3, 106; for chakra opening, 147; daily practice of, 224; emotional health and, 117–18; healing from the past and, 138; how it works, 106–7; mantra-based, 102, 105; physical health and, 51; relationship health and, 180; routines for, 81, 83, 112; thought process and,

meditation (*continued*)
102, 103–5; universal energy and,
105–6
memories, 161, 167–68, 210–11
memory problems, 147
men: communication style of, 171–72;
emotions of, 115; relationship
health and, 155; relationship needs
of, 161–62
metabolic disorders, 144
milk, 66–67, 86
mind-body connection: with food,
70–74, 209; physical and emotional
health, 113–14
mind-body types. *See* doshas (mind-
body types)
moksha (liberation), 153
money: beliefs about, 197–99, 206;
as energy, 196–97, 199–202; fun-
money budget, 205–6; for physical
health, 53–54; physical health and,
196–97; talking about, 204–5, 206
Montessori, Maria, 37
moonlighting, 187
mortgage debt, 196, 202
Mumbai (India), 198

nadi shodhana (alternate-nostril
breathing), 147
Namasté Days, 108
National Public Radio (NPR), 35
Natural by Nature, 61
nature: disconnection from, 80, 109;
emotional rebalancing in, 125–26;
immersion in, for spiritual health,
109; reconnection to, 219–21, 222;
sounds of, in environment, 211–12

navasana (boat pose), 144
neck rolls/circles, 146
neuroassociations, 210
nightmares, 147
9 Steps to Financial Freedom, The
(Orman), 200
90–10 rule, 58, 70
nitpicking, 160, 167
noise, 208–9, 211
Nonviolent Communication (Rosenberg), 122, 172–73
Norwegian University of Science and
Technology, 107
Nyad, Diana, 35

obesity, 1, 142
occupational health: checklist for, 193;
dharma and, 186–89; doshas and,
189–92; exercises, 192–93; job dissatisfaction and, 183–84; meaning
and, 185–87; perspective shifting
for, 184–85. *See also* financial
health; jobs
occupational stress, 183–84
oils, unhealthy, 67–68, 91
oils, Vata-specific, 85–86
online dating, 179
online food sources, 56
Organic Valley, 61
Orman, Suze, 200, 202
osteoarthritis, 51
overachievement, 38–39
overeating, 227
overweight, 1
Oxford University, 109–10

padmasana (lotus flexion), 143
painting, 124

past, the: chakras as healing from, 139–48, 149; checklist for, 149; exercises, 133, 134, 148; imagery from, 213–14; learning lessons from, 137–38, 148, 149; reasons behind, 134–37; relationship failures in, 158; remaining stuck in, 131; stories from, 131–34, 149; taking responsibility for, 136–37

patience, 137–38, 152

peak experiences, 37

pelvic rocks, 143

Perfect Health (Chopra), xviii

perfectionism, 190–91, 218

pessimism, 143

physical health: Ayurvedic nutrition plan, 57–70; checklist for health, 91–92; daily routines for, 80–86, 92; emotional health and, 113–14; exercises, 90–91; fatigue and, 57; financial situation and, 196–97, 206; food quality and, 49–52, 71; laziness and, 55–56; money for, 53–54; physical exercise for, 86–91, 92; in rural areas, 55–56; significant others and, 54–55; taking responsibility for, 51–57; time for, 52–53. *See also* Ayurvedic nutrition plan

physician-patient relationship: author's experience, 29, 30–31; modern Western, 29–30

phytonutrients, 67

Pitta dosha (fire principle) / Pitta types, 23–24; eating awareness guidelines for, 72; emotional rebalancing specific to, 125–26; environmental health for, 218; financial health and, 197; imbalances in, 75, 115–16, 124–25, 175; occupational health for, 190–91; physical exercise routines specific to, 89–90; relationship health and, 174–75; symptom plans for, 31

Pitta-pacifying diet, 66

Pitta-specific diet, 77

Pitta times, 81–83

plank pose, 144

plants, 216

plow pose, 146

portion control, 72

poverty consciousness, 197–98, 200

prakruti (true nature): occupational health and, 189; test for determining, 15–22; as unchangeable, 25–26. *See also* doshas (mind-body types)

prana (life force/vitality), 68–69, 79–80, 139

pranayama (yogic breathing techniques), 142

prayer, 52, 107, 214

prescription medications, 225

present moment, living in, 110, 156–58

preventive medicine, 12–13

Primordial Sound Meditation, 102

produce, organic, 60–61

professional help, 138, 226

pungent (food taste type), 62, 65, 77–78

radiation therapy, 225

radio, 208, 212

rage, 116

ram (mantra), 144

reclining butterfly pose, 143

relationship health: balance and,
    155–59; characteristics of, 159–66,
    180; checklist for, 180–81; commu-
    nication skills for, 156, 163–65, 169,
    170–73, 180; desirable relationship
    creation, 176–78; doshas and,
    173–76, 181; emotional responsi-
    bility and, 118; exercises, 166–69;
    financial debt and, 196, 203; inti-
    mate, finding, 178–80, 181; self-love
    as foundation of, 151–54, 156, 180
relationships: abusive, 138; acceptance
    in, 160, 167; acceptance of current
    state, 156–58; authentic expression
    in, 163–65, 169; balance through,
    155–59; blame assignment in,
    162–63, 168; compassionate com-
    munication in, 170–73, 180; desir-
    able, creating, 176–78; dosha effects
    on, 173–76, 181; gender-differing
    needs in, 161–62, 168; gratitude
    in, 165–66, 169; growth in, 163,
    169; intimate, 154, 157–59, 178–80,
    181; laughter in, 162, 168; learning
    lessons from, 157; love as dynamic
    exchange in, 153; love as uncon-
    ditional in, 159–60, 167; memory
    creation in, 161, 167–68; nitpicking
    in, 160, 167; searching for, 157–59;
    touch in, 160–61, 167; unnourish-
    ing, letting go of, 176; vulnerability
    in, 164
religion, 93, 94, 200, 201
Religions, Values, and Peak-
    Experiences (Maslow), 37
resistance training, 87
retirement funds, 204

right action, 107–12, 229–31
rishis (sages), 14
Robbins, Anthony, 130, 204
root chakra (muladhara), 142–43
Rosenberg, Marshall, 122, 172–73
routine: Ayurveda and, 12, 49; new-
    ness in, for environmental health,
    219–21; for physical health, 80–86,
    92
rural areas, health food stores in,
    55–56

sadness, 116
salty (food taste type), 62, 64, 77–78
salutation pose, 234, 239
Sanskrit terms, glossary of, 243–45
satiation, eating and, 72–73
sattvic (healing) foods, 66–67
savings, emergency, 196, 204
sciatica, 142
Screen-Free Week, 220
self, 144
self-awareness, 138
self-expression, 145
self-healing, 145
self-love, 145, 151–54, 156, 180
self-sufficiency, 153–55
sensory input, for environment, 222;
    smells, 210–11; sounds, 211–12;
    tactile, 212–13; tastes, 209; unneces-
    sary, minimization of, 208–9, 211,
    212; visual imagery, 213–15
sexual chakra (svadhisthana), 143–44
sexual dysfunction, 143
Shakespeare, William, 185, 186
sham (mantra), 147
shame, 162–63, 168
shoulder stands, 146

showers, 85–86

sight, sense of, 213–15

significant others, physical health and, 54–55

silence, 208–9, 212

Simmons, Richard, xvii

Simon, David, 70, 100, 165, 173

singles groups, 179

sivasana, 143

sky reaching in equestrian pose, 235, 238

sky-reaching pose, 234, 238, 239

sleep: meditation and, 102, 107; routines for, 82–86, 209; space for, 83

smells, in environment, 210–11

smiling, 110

smoking, 226–27

snacks, 84

social conditioning, 41, 44–45, 97–99

social media, 220

solar plexus chakra (*manipura*), 144

sore throat, 146

sound, 145; in environment, 211–12

sour (food taste type), 62, 64, 77–78

space (*akasha*), 15, 76, 146, 215–16, 222

space, for sleep, 83

Space-Clearing Commitment (exercise), 216–17

spirituality/spiritual health: checklist for, 112; defined, 93–95, 112; exercises, 101; internal dialogue and, 100–101, 112; intuition and, 96–97, 107, 112; meditation for, 102–7, 112; religion vs., 93, 94; as right action, 107–12; self-love and, 152; social/cultural conditioning and, 97–99; third-eye chakra as source of, 146;

witnessing awareness and, 99–101, 107

spiritual self, finding, 95–97

spiritual superiority, 147

standing bow pose, 145

stiff neck, 146

stories, 131–34, 149

Stories from Your Past, The (exercise), 133

stress: environment and, 214; financial health and, 196; occupational, 183–84

stroke, 1

student loan debt, 196, 204

success, in Western society, 38–39

Sun Salutations, 81, 233–39

surgery, 225; Ayurveda and, 12

sweet (food taste type), 62, 64, 77–78

sweeteners, artificial, 68

Sydney University (Australia), 107

symptom plans, 31–32

Taittiriya Samhita, 232

Taking Inventory of Your Relationship Using the Twelve Traits (exercise), 166–69

Taking Stock of Your Beliefs about Money (exercise), 198–99

taste types, 61–66, 209

Teilhard de Chardin, Pierre, 93, 94

television, 208, 209, 212, 220, 227

Teresa, Mother, 151

texting, 171

third-eye chakra (*ajna*), 146–47

thought(s): control over, 115; meditation and, 102, 103–5; observing, 99–101, 107, 165

thousand-petal lotus chakra (*saha-swara*), 147–48
throat chakra (*vishuddha*), 145–46
thyroid problems, 146
time, for physical health, 52–53
tithing, 201
touch, 110–11, 160–61, 167, 212–13
touch therapy, 12
toxins: emotional, 116–17; past impressions as, 139
Transcendental Meditation, 102, 107
travel, 219
triggers, emotional, 122–23, 227
trust, 45
Tumblr, 220
TV Turn-Off Week, 220
Twitter, 220

ujjayi yogic breathing technique, 146
ulcers, 144, 196
United States: calorie focus in, 59; debt in, 196, 202; disconnection from nature in, 80; goal orientation in, 44–45; physical exercise needed in, 87; poverty consciousness in, 197–98, 200–201; preventable disease rates in, 1; work hours in, 183
University College London, 183
uterine problems, 143

vam (mantra), 143
Vata dosha (wind principle)/Vata types, 22–23; eating awareness guidelines for, 71–72; emotional rebalancing specific to, 123–24; environmental health for, 213,

217–18; financial health and, 197; imbalances in, 74–75, 115, 116, 123, 174; occupational health for, 189–90; physical exercise routines specific to, 89; relationship health and, 174; symptom plans for, 31
Vata-pacifying diet, 66
Vata-specific diet, 76–77
Vata-specific oils, 85–86
Vata tea, 86
Vata times, 81–83
Vedanta, 135, 146
vegan diet, 224–25
vegetables, 67
vibration, 145
victim consciousness, 135–36
vikruti (current state), 26
violence, 142
visual imagery, 213–15
visualization, 47, 142, 147, 179
Vital Farms, 61
voicemail, 171
volunteering, 221
vulnerability, 164

water (*jala*), 15, 76
water, in Ayurvedic nutrition plan, 69–70, 73, 84
Ways You Can Live Outside Your Boxes (exercise), 221
Weil, Andrew, 208
wellness: personal control over, 2, 3; responsibility shifting for, 2–3. *See also* physical health
Western medicine: author's experience, 29–31; Ayurveda vs., 28–29;

goal orientation in, 44–45; physical health and, 52

Western society: self-sufficiency concept in, 153–55; success as defined in, 38–39

white-noise machines, 212

wholeness, principle of, 3–5, 12, 158, 232

Wisnecki, Leonard, 30–31

women: communication style of, 171–72; emotions of, 115; job-related stress in, 183; relationship health and, 155; relationship needs of, 161–62; working, 195

wonder, experiencing, 109

Yajur Veda, 232

yoga: Ayurveda and, 12; chakras and, 142; for creative/sexual chakra (*svadhisthana*), 143–44; for crown chakra (*sahaswara*), 147–48; hatha, 88–89; for heart chakra (*anahata*), 145; hot, 89–90; for root chakra (*muladhara*), 143; routines for, 81, 88–89; for solar plexus chakra (*manipura*), 144; Sun Salutations, 233–39; for third-eye chakra (*ajna*), 147; for throat chakra (*vishuddha*), 146

Your Commitment to Yourself (exercise), 9

Your Dosha-Specific Eating Plan (exercise), 78–79

Your Emotional Healing Plan (exercise), 127–30

Your New Reality (exercise), 134

Your Three Lessons to Take to Your Fulfilling Future (exercise), 148

YouTube, 220

yum (mantra), 145

ABOUT *the* AUTHOR

Michelle S. Fondin is owner of the Ayurvedic Path Yoga and Wellness Studio, which she founded in 2008, where she practices as an Ayurvedic lifestyle counselor and as a yoga and meditation teacher. She holds a Vedic Master certificate from the Chopra Center, has worked with Dr. Deepak Chopra at Chopra Center events teaching yoga and meditation, and currently writes for Chopra.com. She's a member of the National Ayurvedic Medical Association, the Association of Ayurvedic Professionals of North America, and Yoga Alliance. When Michelle isn't writing or teaching, she likes to spend time playing with her three children, running with her boyfriend, eating Indian food, and salsa dancing. You can learn more on her website, www.michellefondin.com/about-michelle/.

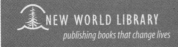